To See Another Sunrise...

How To Overcome Anything, One Day At A Time

To DEBORAH

Jim Morrison

By Jim Morrison,
Stage 4 cancer survivor

To See Another Sunrise...
How To Overcome Anything, One Day At A Time
Jim Morrison

Production Design: Jeff Rowley
Editor: David Kilmer

ISBN 13: 978-1480287693
ISBN 10: 1480287695

Dedication

To my 9th grade sweetheart, best friend and mother of my children, my wife Sandi. I love you with all my heart. To daughter Kym, Jimmy and their boys, to son Jeff and Stephanie. To Sandi's brother Gary and his wife Julie, a breast cancer survivor. To my sister Janet, my sister-in-law Joan, and all my "in-laws and outlaws." I couldn't have done it without you.

Contents

Foreword

Why do I like practicing as an oncologist/hematologist – a physician who treats cancer and blood disorders? When I first fell in love with oncology, I was still a medical student. Serendipitously, I did my summer internship in oncology rather than cardiology at the university clinic in Gottingen, Germany, and the wonderful physicians at the oncology service introduced me to the exciting field of cancer care and research. Later, while I pursued a career in academic medicine, research and the desire to find new ways of treating cancer and blood disorders were my motivations.

Over the last 16 years, I practiced in beautiful Northern Idaho. I am sure like many other oncologists, there have been many times when I have asked the same question: why do I love practicing oncology? I know the same reasons that made me fall in love initially – research and innovative thinking – are still important, but there is another deeper reason: meeting amazing people like Jim Morrison.

A diagnosis of cancer is a life-altering event for most individuals, their families and friends. There is an extraordinary courage and strength that I witness with each patient and their journey with this disease. I am the most happy and fulfilled when I can be of help during their journey with my skills, knowledge and chosen profession.

Jim Morrison's diagnosis is not unusual; if anything, it unfortunately remains a relatively common presentation of lung cancer and is considered incurable. The involvement of the pericardial sac, the lining that covers the heart, is associated with an even poorer outcome in clinical studies. However, what is unique and well worth reading in this book is the amalgamation of his inner strength, his family and community support, his mindset towards the disease, and his adaptation to the treatment and effects of the disease and the science of cancer biology and medicine.

Unfortunately, not all individuals with advanced cancer have or will have the outcome that Jim Morrison has until we can better understand cancer, a plethora of diseases each with many different biological subtypes and a need for different approach.

Jim's story is about hope, adaptability and inner strength, which are, in my opinion, crucial for any individual dealing with a difficult disease like cancer. Through the years, I have observed that the patients with this kind of outlook have had better outcomes whether it is clinically or emotionally.

This is Jim's personal story with a difficult cancer, but there are many good lessons, tips and anecdotes that will undoubtedly help other individuals with similar difficult problems and give a different perspective of surviving cancer. Even physicians will get a glimpse into the thoughts of a cancer survivor with a good sense of humor and wit.

I also hope that through his book and the type of treatment he is still receiving, a personalized cancer treatment designed to treat a very specific subtype of common lung cancer, readers will appreciate the importance of research into cancer biology and clinical trials that will allow physicians to ask questions and develop better treatments for individuals with these difficult diseases. Also, his treatment had many "outside the box" approaches that required a close relationship and trust between Jim and his medical team, which is not possible in an environment of cookie-cutter medicine.

I thoroughly enjoyed reading this book. I recommend it for everybody, whether a cancer survivor, a patient with a chronic illness, their family, friends or physicians. I do not think this is a recipe or should be read as such on how to survive cancer. Instead, I see it as a story that exemplifies wisdom, strength, values and determination that we, human beings, have. With hope and adaptation, we have a chance to overcome many adversities like my dear friend Jim did.

–Haluk Tezcan, MD

Editor's Preface

For a guy who's supposed to be dead right now, Jim Morrison lives life at quite a pace. Our meetings are always high-energy affairs in which I do my best to keep up with his enthusiastic approach to everything.

In many ways Jim's response to cancer has made him stronger than ever: as a family man, as a counselor for those who he calls his fellow "cancer warriors," and as a spokesman for the Kootenai Cancer Center that helped save his life.

Since his terrifying diagnosis he continues to reach one huge milestone after the next. He is living life faster than he can write it down. Really, the final chapter of this book is unfinished – because Jim continues to experience it day by day. It's written in the sparkle in his eye, the confidence in his stride, the giant grin on his face.

My new friend Jim is living proof that you, too, can do the impossible… One day at a time.

–David Kilmer,
Editor

Author's Preface

On a cold January day in 2004, I learned just how fragile life can be.

A duck hunting trip led to the hospital, which led to a diagnosis of Stage 4 cancer in my lungs that had spread to the sac around my heart. It was a death sentence.

And yet... *I survived.* In the dark hours right after my diagnosis, I found hope. And through the countless medical treatments that ultimately saved my life, I found reasons to live – the first dance at my daughter's wedding, the birth of my first grandson, my son's college graduation, and even helping others with cancer.

This is my story – the good, the bad and the ugly. As you will find, I am a guy who speaks his mind. If you have received a cancer diagnosis, or are a family member of someone with cancer, this book is for you. If you are fighting an addiction, or any other life-altering challenge, or maybe just need a new appreciation of life's blessings, it's for you, too.

I wrote this book to tell you how I survived, and even more, how I found hope.

Cancer changed my life – for the better.

I wish the same for you.

–Jim Morrison, 2012

What Cancer Cannot Do

It cannot cripple love
It cannot shatter hope
It cannot corrode faith

It cannot destroy peace
It cannot kill friendship
It cannot suppress memories

It cannot silence courage
It cannot invade the soul
It cannot steal eternal life

It cannot conquer the spirit

–Author Unknown

"Courage is not the absence of fear, but the conquest of it."

–Unknown

Introduction

Welcome! This is cancer warrior Jim Morrison, inviting you to climb aboard this crazy ride I've been on for eight years… and counting.

This is the story of an average guy who takes on one of the toughest diseases – stage 4 lung cancer. The survival rate is very low. But guess what? I have lived to complete some impossible goals. Now I am eager to share my hard-fought victories with you.

Why did I write this book? Because I want you to know that the courage of a person is gauged by how much it takes to discourage them. And I want you to hold onto hope after the heartbreak of being told you have cancer. *I won – and you can too.*

I pay my dues each and every day for surviving my battle against cancer. I could have chosen an easier way. I could have given up and allowed my foe to take its course. But no, I had to fight. I want you to know, my fellow cancer warrior, that I fought against all odds – and so will you. *What odds? What fight? What cancer?* Let them call us crazy. In the meantime, you and I are going to tackle the impossible together!

I am a former heating and cooling contractor who lives in gorgeous North Idaho. With each amazing birthday – 59 of them at this writing – I continue to defy the medical odds. I am forever happily married to my 9th grade sweetheart Sandi. We've just celebrated our 40th anniversary. Later, I will share how cheating in spelling gained me my best friend for life.

You will meet the rest of my wonderful family as we go: My

daughter Kym is married to my son-in-law Jimmy, with three great boys, Austin, Byron and Carter. My son Jeff is married to my daughter-in-law Stephanie. We have ordered a granddaughter from them! My wife's brother Gary and his wife Julie, a breast cancer survivor, have two girls and live close to us. They currently own and operate my former air conditioning and heating business, which cancer stole from me, as you will see.

My extended family includes my sister Janet and her three boys and their families in Oregon, and my wonderful mother-in-law Mama, who is sharp as a tack at 88, and Sandi's sister Joan. I have many more great in-laws (and outlaws!). For all of them, I am grateful.

The way I see it, the reason I'm living and breathing today is because of faith, family and medical facilities. Each played a huge role during my war with cancer.

My medical professionals – every one of them – are absolutely incredible. From day one, I have been blessed to be cared for by the new state-of-the-art Kootenai Cancer Center here in North Idaho. Every positive milestone I reach, I've celebrated with my oncologist Dr. Tezcan and his two wonderful nurses, Jennifer and Patricia. They have watched my family grow, and with me they've relished the happiness I feel.

Our world today feeds on a celebrity culture of entertainment and gossip. That's not what I'm offering you. This is a true story – I am living it every day. I want to be a part of your battle with cancer. I would like to think of myself as a mentor. If you'll allow me, I'd like to go with you step by step on your own journey.

I want to encourage you with the hope that extended my life. Yes, cancer kills, but it has not killed me yet, nor has it you! Yes, cancer can affect every person differently. But I also know this fact: that true faith and courage is the same yesterday, today and forever. If you are beginning your cancer journey, there will be plenty of pain, suffering and "what if's" – along with joy and sorrow – to come. But let me encourage you with this: At my next checkup, if my scans are clear and blood marker is good, I will have six years of remission as of 2013. Remember, my initial diagnosis was six months to live.

Throughout my battle with cancer, I've often been told, "Jim, you are as stubborn as a mule." It reminds me of a story that helps me every day. I know it will help you.

There once was a farmer who owned an old mule. One day, the mule fell into the farmer's well. The farmer heard the mule praying, or whatever mules do when they fall into wells. After assessing the situation, the farmer sympathized with the mule, but decided that neither the mule nor the well was worth the trouble of saving. Instead, he enlisted his neighbors to help haul dirt to bury the old mule in the well and put him out of his misery.

As dirt began to fall onto his back, the mule was hysterical with fear. But as the farmer and his neighbors continued to shovel, a thought struck the old mule: Every time a shovel load of dirt landed on his back, *he would shake it off and step up!* This he did, blow after blow. *"Shake it off and step up... shake it off and step up...shake it off and step up!"* He repeated it often to encourage himself. No matter how painful the blows, or how distressing the situation seemed, the mule fought panic and just kept right on *shaking it off and stepping up!* It wasn't long before the old mule, battered and exhausted, stepped triumphantly over the wall of the well. What seemed like it would bury him actually helped him…all because of the manner in which he handled his adversity.

No matter what cancer sends you, I want you to promise not to be discouraged. I want you to *shake it off* and keep going. As a cancer warrior, the best way to predict your future is to help create it. Set a goal, and achieve that goal. Then set a new goal.

By shaking it off, and stepping up, I have lived to give my beautiful daughter's hand in marriage. I have lived to hold my new baby grandchildren. With that mindset, I have now lived long enough to see my son graduate… and then ask his girlfriend to marry him. I lived long enough to actually perform in my son's ceremony – at a wedding I should never had attended! For a man whose life has been measured in hours and days, these are amazing milestones, indeed.

And I have also been hunting. Now for some of you, that might not mean much. For a hunting nut like me, it means the world. To realize how passionate I am about this sport, you should know that in the midst of the pain and confusion of early cancer, when I needed a port put into my shoulder for chemotherapy, I made sure to ask my doctors to put it in my left shoulder. That's because I wanted to make sure I could continue duck hunting with my son – and I needed my right shoulder to hold my gun! Later, when I was so weak I could not stand, my friends even pushed me to the marshes in my wheelchair. I remember them taking my picture, and thinking, "They never take pictures of me hunting. Why are they doing it now?" Then I realized why.

I want you to find what matters most to you in life. I want you to hold fast to that through the tough times. And I want you to beat your cancer so you can get back to enjoying your life.

I was hunting ducks when I first felt the icy hands of cancer on my shoulders.

And I was hunting ducks again, seven years later in October 2011, when I celebrated my freedom and newfound strength and health.

I want to share that joyful duck hunt with you because I want you to know how it feels to be free again. I want you to know that no matter the struggle, you can persevere. You can live to see your dreams come true.

For me, that realization came most recently as I lay in my hunting blind in an Alberta, Canada pea field, hunting with my boy Jeff. For the past few years, he had said "Dad, how cool would it be to go to Canada together and get all three types of geese on one hunt?" And my health had been the barrier. Now, with Dr. Tezcan's blessing, we hoped to realize my son's goal. As I gave thanks for that moment, I realized it is enough simply to be alive, to smell the fields, watch the light gradually brighten, hear the excitement in the other hunters' voices...

What a beautiful morning it is. The sun is now throwing shooting light over us. I look out through my blind lid to watch a hundred mallard ducks sail over our blinds at ten feet and land in the decoys. Feeling comfortable, they begin feeding and walking toward our blinds. What a sight! I love to watch wildlife do their thing undisturbed. As the geese start to work our spread, it spooks the ducks. The sound of that many ducks taking off is so cool. Circling right over me so close that if I raised my blind lid I could hit them, the air off their wings against my face, oh what a dream come true. When I was in the infusion room doing my chemotherapy, I never dreamed anything could feel so good again.

Now there are so many geese, and their calls are so loud, that I have to yell at Jeff: "WOW, THIS IS INCREDIBLE!" And he still can't hear me, even from five feet away. As the number of birds continues to build I can see snow geese, specklebelly geese and Canada geese, along with three or four species of ducks, flying up over our blinds. Some Canada geese have landed in our decoys along with the hundreds of ducks. The sound – and the sheer number of birds – is unbelievable. What an experience to witness this with my hunting buddies who have pulled for me since I was first diagnosed with cancer.

Anticipation builds until the time is just right, then Jeff is up and shooting, and the rest of us are too, and there is an indescribable flurry of shotguns, birds and then of tears on my face, as I watch my son confirm not one, not two, but three kinds of geese for his hunt. This moment has only been a picture in my mind until today. As I extended to my son, not the gentleman's handshake, but instead a mighty hug, I was here – and cancer could not take me away.

A month after that waterfowl trip, I packed my truck and headed back to Canada for a deer hunt.

"But Jim," you say, "you have stage 4 lung cancer." Yes, you're right.

"But you had three hard years of chemotherapy." Right again.

"You have deep vein thrombosis – blood clots in your legs." Yes, I do.

"You have been sick seven years and still take a pill and give yourself an injection every morning." So what? I'm alive! I admit that my cancer might kill me someday, but it won't be today. Tomorrow, I'm going hunting.

You ask, "Jim, what if your cancer comes back and you die?" I can tell you that I am ready. Just so you know, I prepared my own funeral service right after I was diagnosed, explaining the whole thing to my wife Sandi. I take comfort in the fact that my family will celebrate the fact that God extended my life to complete my work here and to enjoy life's finest moments with family and friends. Now my goal is to help you find new life in the midst of this most relentless of diseases.

I wrote this book to encourage you that tomorrow's sunrise is for you. And not only for you, but for all cancer warriors and anyone else who struggles with living just one more day. Living for today is good, and living long enough for tomorrow is even better. But live for next month… and you might just find yourself hunting in a pea field seven years later.

My real life story will encourage, scare, make you laugh, cry and piss you off. But to that I say; "Talk to the picture of my beautiful Alberta deer." It's a photo that should have never been taken, if cancer had had its way.

Hey there, cancer warrior, "Got goals?" The most important thing about a goal is simply having one. I need you to fight, I need you to keep focused on the day by day through this toughest part of your life. Welcome the refreshing wind of victory. Even when the odds don't look good, you need those goals. Don't let cancer take them away.

I love you, my fellow cancer warrior. I know very well your every thought and pain. Thank you for letting me share my story with you.

Someday in the future, I will read yours.

CHAPTER 1
Taken Captive By Cancer

It was a cold Idaho day when I first felt cancer's icy touch. We were loading up the boat to go waterfowl hunting, one of my favorite things to do. A January snowstorm had buried the driveway, so I grabbed a shovel and began to dig. For some reason, I really struggled to catch my breath, becoming more exhausted with every futile stab at the snow.

"Hey, Jimbo, too much for you, old man?" said my boy Jeff, using his affectionate nickname for me.

"Just pacing myself." I gasped for air and leaned on my shovel.

I'm a guy who's spent his life at a physical job and in the outdoors, and I'm rarely outworked by anyone. Something was wrong.

My brother-in-law Gary drove up with the truck, and we hooked up the boat, drove to one of our favorite hunting spots near Lake Coeur d'Alene, and set up the blinds and decoys as the snow continued to fall.

"What the heck is wrong with me today?" I asked myself. "I should not be this tired."

Those who know me know I'm not a quitter. And when I wanted to give up the hunt and return to the truck, my hunting partners realized that we'd better pack it up and head straight for home. My wife Sandi was shocked by the way I looked.

"Oh my goodness, are you okay? You're as white as a ghost. You get to bed now."

I felt awful. As I struggled to climb the stairs to my bedroom, I was gasping for air and my legs were beginning to hurt. Sure, I was exhausted from a very busy week at work, but I knew something else wasn't right – I just didn't have a clue what it was.

The next morning I wasn't any better. "Give me another day, I'll be alright," I told Sandi. She was having none of that, so off to the emergency room we went. After we took a series of tests and lab work, I was relieved to get back and rest at home, in front of the football game I was missing on TV. I would soon discover that was the least of my worries.

SIGNS OF TROUBLE

It turned out my gallbladder was failing, and so I underwent surgery. I knew I was fortunate to be in the capable hands of the world-class medical facility at Kootenai Health in Coeur d'Alene. I thought I'd get that surgery over and get back to my life. But I wasn't doing so well.

As I lay in the hospital, the doctors continued to run tests, including ultrasound, X-rays and CT scans. My legs were burning and hurting, and I couldn't walk. I was so nauseous that when a lab tech came into my room to draw blood, the smell of her perfume set me into uncontrollable vomiting spasms. It was so hard to breathe that I felt like an elephant was sitting on my chest.

I felt myself becoming weaker and weaker. When my longtime family doctor, Susan Daugharty-Fowler, came into the room crying, I knew it would be the worst kind of news.

With Sandi by my side, my doctor, with tears in her eyes, gave us those words that will be burned into my mind forever:

"The CT scan shows a tumor in the top third of your left lung. The X-rays show massive amounts of fluid in both lungs and around your heart. We need to extract this fluid right now to relieve the pressure."

Almost immediately, there were five doctors in my hospital room, and they were all very busy. My doctor asked Sandi to call family members and bring them to the hospital as soon as possible.

Sandi left my room hysterical with fear that I would die before she returned.

My doctor bent down close to my ear, tears still in her eyes. "We have maybe two hours to handle this or we could lose you. Your body is shutting down. Hang in there, Jim."

She gave me a hug, and then I was wheeled out of there at break-neck speed, down to the ICU emergency room where they sat me up to remove the fluid from my lungs. The process was neither pretty nor slow. It was obvious that it was a life-and-death situation. But with the fluid gone, the elephant had been removed, and I could breathe again.

I remember resting back in my own hospital bed, with my two-hour death sentence expired. I was overwhelmed with joy that I'd made it – not just for me, but more importantly for my family and their future. For the moment, I rested in sweet peace, with a new lease on life and my wife at my side.

But I was far from okay.

THE TERRIBLE NEWS

The new day brought a new procedure. I remember watching on a TV screen as a doctor ran a probe down through an artery in my leg and up near my heart. There, he installed an inferior vena cava filter (IVC filter). The idea was to prevent the blood clots now discovered in both legs from traveling to where they could do any more damage. Wow, how fragile that can make a guy feel.

It was now January 12, 2004, day number nine of my "one night in the hospital." By now, the pathology report was ready on the fluid removed from my lungs. My family doctor planned to give us the results. I wished for the best, but I prepared my mind for bad news. I was not setting myself up, just dealing with facts.

My entire family was now gathered all around my bed waiting. I felt grateful that I was still alive to be here with them. Whatever this doctor's report brought, I felt blessed by the love and support of my family. Time would later reveal just how important this support would prove to be.

You could cut the fear with a knife. The anxiety built to a peak when Dr. Daugherty-Fowler walked into my room. We said our good mornings, and she introduced another doctor, oncologist Haluk Tezcan. Then she began crying, and the reality began to set in. Dr. Tezcan told us that the results were "Bad, very bad."

The silence was broken by crying and exclamations of shock. Bracing myself for the rest of his report, I reached for my wife's hand, the same hand I had reached to for most of my life, and collected myself to ask the doctor to continue.

"The findings show stage 4 lung cancer which has metastasized to the pericardial sac around your heart," he said. "This is rare, and usually does not respond to treatment as well." After that came some more technical information that I was sure only my nurse daughter understood and could later break down for the rest of us. Again, silent worry filled the room.

The question had to be asked – the hardest words I have ever spoken.

"How long do I have to live?" I asked the doctor. "I want it straight, no nonsense."

He drew a deep breath and gave me my death sentence.

"Based on my experience and past reported cases of the disease with no response to treatment? Six months," he said.

"And if you respond to treatment and have no side effects? A year and a half."

Lying there, looking into the eyes of everyone I cared for, I felt helpless and empty. Everyone was so stunned by the news that it was like they were frozen. Could anything good come out of this? Only time would tell.

THE GRIM TALLY

It turns out I had several serious health challenges. The stage 4 (metastatic) non-small cell lung cancer had spread to the pericardium, the sac around my heart. It was so close that radiation therapy or surgical removal were both out of the question. I needed chemotherapy.

I also had disseminated intravascular coagulation, or DIC, a clotting of small blood vessels throughout the body, and often a precursor to massive organ failure. I continued to have cardiac tamponade, a compression of the heart that occurs when blood or fluid builds up in the space between the myocardium (heart muscle) and the pericardium (outer covering sac of the heart). I would undergo surgery for this, as well as a separate surgery for the fluid in my lungs. All told, Jim Morrison was just about a dead man. But not yet!

CONFRONTING DEATH

At 3 a.m. on January 13, 2004, I was a desperate and broken man, staring at the ceiling of the ICU. My dear wife was at my side, passed out in a very uncomfortable chair from emotional exhaustion. For me, sleeping was out of the question that night. My mind raced to sort through all the bad news.

I couldn't disengage my brain from reminding me that I was very sick, and that I might have only a short time to live. My entire being feared this fact to the point of complete helplessness. My sick and nervous stomach was in turmoil, and there was no comfortable position for my body to rest. A hollow and powerless feeling penetrated to the very marrow of my bones. My body had been taken captive by the one thing I feared the most. My once bright future was now severely dimmed by one word: CANCER.

As I wrestled this overwhelming black cloud over me, I felt like I was trying to bail water from the Titanic. Feeling desperate, I reached for the only book I'd brought from home, my Bible. I didn't really know where or even why I wanted to read. On its own, the book invited me into the pages of the Book of Daniel.

I was so weak I didn't have the strength to hold the Bible, so I had to prop it up on the pillows. I begin reading slowly, paying attention to every word. By the end of chapter 6 it became clear to me, in my desperate hour, that this very moment was no coincidence.

I felt that divine intervention was asking me to make a decision. With nothing but my life, now riddled with cancer, to offer, I became willing to accept the truth.

As the new day dawned, I woke my wife and shared with her,

through my tears, the realization that had just taken place in our room. And from that first moment when I read those words from Daniel, lying broken on my deathbed, right on through my tremendous struggle with illness and to my existence in remission today, they are my strength, my encouragement and my new life.

SURRENDERING MY SELF

The biggest thing I learned from my experience in the ICU was surrender. If I wanted to survive cancer, I had to let God be God and me be me. If I truly wanted peace in my life, I could not remain in control.

Faith is something you must put to work. For example, if you need light in your room, you need to flip the light switch. The light bulb won't shine until you make the choice to use it. For anything we confront, the self-made attitude is dangerous. We all need help – a higher power, if you will. On our own is never enough.

It was very difficult for me to accept that I was not in control. I realized I was going to have to surrender myself and get out of my own way to get healed. I raised the white flag and asked for help from God, the medical staff and my family. I resolved to turn the switch on and live by the new light shining within. I was amazed by how much bigger and brighter things suddenly looked without my self-doubt blocking the light.

This was the hardest, and the most important thing of all. I felt that if I was not right inside, nothing I attempted during this scariest part of my life would amount to anything. I didn't have time for a second chance. It was time now to choose who I wanted to control my life, at least what I had left of it. The self-made Jim Morrison died that early morning. But my new life, even with cancer, had just begun.

HAPPY TO BE HOME

After 14 days in the hospital, and many tests, scans, x-rays, consultations and prayers, I was released to go home. I can't tell you what a thrill that was, being wheeled to the door amid hugs, handshakes and tears.

Believe it or not, my departure was with mixed emotion. Oh, how I wanted to go home, but how do you say "thank you" to the incredible medical staff who just saved your life? These wonderful people had helped my family and me through a very stressful two weeks, and their passion and compassion comforted us all.

I was conscious of the fact that I could very well have been horizontal, heading in a very different direction. I was overcome with the grace of God.

I knew how close I'd come to dying. Leaving there that day, I felt in my soul that something was about to take place in my life. Good or bad, I was not sure. But I had a hunch that this extended life had been given, not just to me, but to others. But to whom? And why?

THE REAL TEST

It was good to be home again. Wow! What an experience, going from life to death and back to life again. I made myself comfortable in my new La-Z-Boy recliner chair, a new gift from my dear family. This is where I pretty much lived. I had to keep my legs up all day, and walking was still very tiring and painful. There were too many stairs for me to go to our bedroom.

Some days, my legs and ankles would swell to twice their normal size. We had fun setting golf balls in the divots that you could indent on my legs, a symptom called pitting edema. Really fun, right? Adjusting to this new way of living was difficult. But as I spent countless hours every day and night in my reclining chair, I had an opportunity to reflect back on the whole picture. So many things had happened so quickly, and now I had the time to sort through it all and try to make sense of this whirlwind ride.

Looking back at my life, I realized I had experienced pain and sorrow, joy and sadness, good and bad. I had confronted the best and worst in myself, and mourned the death of others. We all have – it's a part of life.

I must admit that when I heard the word cancer, the thought of death was immediate. My time had come to get ready to die. *Well, just wait a minute,* I told myself now. *You can go that route if you want. But I am either too stupid to know you can't beat cancer or smart enough to know you can, with help.*

The real test was still ahead. In two weeks, my chemotherapy treatments would begin. I was sure a new adjustment was coming soon.

A LIFE WORTH LIVING

I am fortunate to be blessed with an amazing family. When all my hope seemed lost, it was the thought of them that kept me going.

Without my family's love, help and support, I would not be here today. My sister drove through a blinding ice storm to be by my side when it counted. My wife's family left everything to be here for us, and they were a tremendous help in this awful time. My family lived, ate, slept and worried every day right outside my hospital room. Every night, some family member would be in the room with me.

My daughter Kym, a registered nurse, would leave her hospital to come directly to mine. She was a great help to break down everything the doctors were telling us. I worried about her because she knew too much. Sometimes I could see it in her eyes, and I would try to remind her to just be my daughter. My son had to leave college to be with us, costing him valuable time and creating hardships.

My sister-in-law, Joan, bless her unselfish heart, devoted her entire day to helping sort through mountains of paperwork, phone calls and scheduling doctor's appointments. She became our personal secretary so that Sandi and I could enjoy whatever time we had left together. Her relentless energy gave me what I needed to survive.

My brother-in-law, Gary, took over my heating and cooling business, making sure customers stayed warm that long Idaho winter while I was confined to my hospital bed, and later my La-Z-Boy recliner at home.

Without Gary, this company I had started from scratch would not have made it. In the blink of an eye, he had the responsibility of a business, his family, his sister's family and my grim diagnosis all thrown on his shoulders. His days were as long and challenging as mine – and we both survived.

And I had another support group, too. The hospital staff became my newest family. What a committed and dedicated group of professionals they were, helping us all the way through our struggle. Without their encouragement – and certainly their incredible care – you would not be reading this story today.

IMPOSSIBLE GOAL #1

It was my family – and maybe my stubborn nature – that I have to blame for "Jim's Impossible Goals." There have been a few along the way. I'd like to share these with you, fellow warrior. You will see how I "made up my mind" (Daniel 1:8) to get there. You will see that you can, too.

My first big impossible goal was giving my daughter's hand in marriage. This was on my mind right after the shock of my fatal diagnosis had sunk in.

You see, my sweet baby Kym planned to be married on July 17, 2004. I was terrified. That was six months away! I had heard the doctor say it: I could be dead by then.

My daughter was incredibly loving and unselfish. Even though her wedding was the biggest event in her young life, she thought even more of my needs. She told me she would move the date up two months earlier so I could attend. She also began to cancel her reservations for flowers, food and reception hall, offering me the money instead for cancer treatments. Amazing!

Sandi and I discussed our options when we could. In the days following a chemotherapy treatment I was always sick, especially days three and four. Some days I'd sleep the whole day, some days I'd feel ill and too weak to talk, and the other days I'd be just plain exhausted from the five-hour infusion treatments.

Over time we came to a decision. I had "made up my mind." I asked Kym to come sit in the chair that's always next to my recliner, and I shared my heart with her.

"Listen," I told her. "Keep your wedding on the day you originally planned, July 17. That's six months away. Kym, please keep that carrot out there. Make me make it. This is my first goal of my extended life and new mindset. I will fight one hour at a time. I WILL be at your wedding and we will have our father-daughter dance."

THE FIRST DANCE

I thought chemotherapy was tough. Try walking your only daughter down the aisle to give her away!

Kym loves flip-flops, so she wore them for the ceremony. Her bridesmaids did too. I wore my shiny and stiff new tux shoes – right up to the start of our walk up the aisle. Kym was very impressed I would dress so formal for her big day. That's when I slipped on black flip-flops for our walk together. FUN! *Alive and having fun. What cancer?*

As we made our way down the center aisle, I noticed almost everyone was crying, like we were. I was so excited to be there, but so not wanting to give my Kym away. I knew Jimmy was great, but she's my baby. One word, "cancer," had almost rendered me helpless, but now four little words, "her mother and I", gave me an inexplicable sense of accomplishment, along with the reality that my baby was now a wife.

I sat down next to Sandi as we shared tears of mixed emotions. As I watched the ceremony, I couldn't help but think how blessed we were, how well "Plan B" had turned out after all, and how something as terrible as cancer could make this evening so special.

It was time for our dance. The long-awaited moment had arrived. This is what I'd pledged to fight for, to be here for.

As I tried to get up from my chair, I felt weak at the knees. Kym slowly walked onto the dance floor. She was radiant and breathtaking. She looked at me through eyes of fear and joy, well aware that I could easily not have been here for this dance.

Meeting my baby girl on that dance floor was beyond any words I know. A powerful feeling overcame the guests. We were in a moment of time only possible by faith, and no one could deny it.

The song began to play: *"I'll Always Be Your Baby"* by Natalie

Grant. I hugged my daughter on her wedding day. I was alive. I'd made it here by living two more hours in the ICU, by living one more day at a time.

My daughter's head on my shoulder gave me new hope. It was a feeling I would never have experienced without cancer. We danced together against all odds, six months after that cold January day when darkness fell heavy on the hearts of the Morrison family. That night I had never seen brighter stars. And my future felt bright, too.

My dad once told me; "Your son is a son 'til he takes a wife. Your daughter is a daughter for the rest of her life." Kym was young and full of life, and by experiencing this night along with her, my family, friends and faith, so was I.

Having the strength to dance with the bride gave me more strength. In that moment, I started a new hourglass. I determined that while I suffered through the next post-chemotherapy days, instead of just watching the sand slowly pour from one place to the next, I would contemplate what goal I could achieve next.

To this day, I thank my God for allowing that unbelievable night. Our picture together on the dance floor adorns the top of the mantle in our home. To this day and forever, I will gain strength from it. And when you hear this story, my friend, my prayer is that you can, too.

HEARTFELT THOUGHTS

Later on, you will read about more of "Jim's Impossible Goals." For now, I want to give you some heartfelt thoughts from my first six months of living with cancer.

The realization that I might never live to see my daughter married was heavy stuff. Welcome to the battle of cancer. My first six months were filled with highs and lows, bigger than I had experienced in fifty years of life. The lows were overwhelming – not only from facing death within, but from seeing in the eyes of my loved ones the fear of losing me. There were not-so-good days; okay, there were horrible days. Sometimes many of them.

My fight was fueled not only by my commitment to Kym, but by the fact that if I died, it would be the most selfish thing I could ever do to my loving family. This is what I thought about for six months. Staring death in the face makes for restlessness. *So much, so little time, how do I do the right things? What are the right things?* My mentor, Don, who you will meet soon in this book, was a tremendous help to me during this time. His experience with cancer was priceless to me. *Who is YOUR mentor?*

These were my high moments: I walked to the bathroom. I answered the phone. I watched a whole football game without one nap. I ate lunch. For a new cancer warrior, those are the highest of highs.

Another high was being able to visit with the great folks who came to see me. When I was on chemotherapy, the windows of quality time were small. The best visits were short ones!

During this time, it was a wonderful experience just to sit at the kitchen table to eat with my family. There were highs I can't explain. There was a feeling that comes up from within: *I can do this!* At the time, I had no clue how. But to feel and to believe that was uplifting. I felt an incredible high from a goodnight kiss from Sandi or her "good job" love tap on my shoulder for another 24-hour victory.

Life was simple, but it was the toughest time I have ever experienced.

My first six months with cancer set the tone for everything that followed. I believe that will be true for you, too. You must deal with every level of your life – spiritual, physical, emotional and mental. The goals you set RIGHT NOW will make all the difference.

When my daughter's wedding and my potential death fell on the same month, I knew I might not survive to see the wedding. I refused that option. That gave me three choices that I kept in front of me, every single day, for those six difficult months:

A. Watch a video of the wedding from my recliner (if I could stay awake).

B. Make it to the wedding, but be unable to do much but sit there.

C. Walk my daughter down the aisle wearing our flip flops for one of my life's most memorable moments.

Any one of these options, on any given day, was correct. But in the end, the best and only goal I would accept came true. That was my first dance with my daughter, the bride.

I love you, my fellow cancer warrior. Let's get to it!

MY FIRST GRANDSON

For a cancer patient, any good news is always welcome. We live under the constant question of *"What if?"* and the expectation of bad news. I will never forget the words of my doctor, "I have good news and very bad news. How do you want me to start?"

When Cabela's outdoor store had their grand opening near my home in Post Falls, Idaho, I was absolutely ecstatic. Even though I couldn't get out of my chair to go, it was good news nonetheless. When new hunting magazines would arrive, I was happy. It was even good news just to see the sunrise. In many ways, my new world had become very simple – I would enjoy good news and adjust to the bad.

With my daughter's wedding accomplished, I needed a new goal. I remembered a saying from my Dad's recovery groups: *If you jump to the top of a curb and fall short, you land in the gutter. But if you shoot for the moon and fall short, you land on a star.*

I decided that hanging on until Christmas was my next goal. And I made it! I had survived nearly a year. What a gift for all of us to celebrate life together. What else could bring more joy? Well, that would be my daughter, announcing during our Christmas celebration that my wife and I were going to be grandparents.

I was so excited with the good news that it carried me for weeks. One day in the infusion room during treatment, however, stark reality hit me. The birth date was predicted for July. Could I make it another six months? What if I didn't, and missed the birth of my first grandchild?

As I watched an ultrasound picture, showing a wonderful healthy baby boy, I decided that nothing would stop me from seeing and holding my newborn grandson. I'd made up my mind!

I marked off the days on the calendar one at a time. Soon I was marking off the months. The wait for this little miracle seemed to crawl by.

And then, wonder of wonders, I was next to my daughter's bed in the maternity room, sometimes standing, sometimes sitting when I ran out of strength. After a year and a half of cancer I was alive, and overjoyed.

I looked at that new life, and I just melted.

I held my grandson in my arms, and through my tears of joy, I looked into his eyes. I kissed his forehead and it infused me with a new sense of power, cutting past the draining fatigue of chemotherapy. Finally, by orders, I had to relinquish my love grip on my new little buddy.

I decided right then and there – I would live long enough to watch him grow into a young man.

This July, 2012, my grandson Byron will be seven years old. I call him "Mr. B." Every time I'm around that little guy, my heart melts. I love him so much. My daughter once brought him to the hospital to see me after one of my surgeries, and holding him, I could feel a newfound strength to live.

How do I thank God for extending my life to include my precious grandson? Could it be the reason you're reading this story? Could my survival encourage you to stay alive, to reach your own goals against all odds? You can't do it vicariously through me. You, and you alone, must seek the faith and power. Find that purpose in your heart and put into action what you know is right. Your life depends on it.

THE GRADUATION

My son was in college when I got sick. Living two hours away made it tough on him. He was always worrying about me and would call every night. Every break he got, he was home in an instant.

He wasn't scheduled to graduate until May of 2007. How much could we ask for here? I had lived long enough to dance with my daughter at her wedding, see the birth of my precious grandson, and now I was asking to watch my only son graduate from college.

I had my moments when all the "What ifs" would overcome me.

But I refused to let them hold me down. I learned to live by faith, but to deal with reality. I knew that the shadow of a dog cannot bite you, nor can the shadow of death kill you. Keep walking! Get out from under the shadow to where there's light. You can do this. You must!

In the summer of 2004, my son and I hatched a brilliant plan to spend that fall season hunting waterfowl. There were only a few bugs to work out:

A. I had stage 4 lung cancer and was doing very intense chemo.
B. I couldn't walk very far or breathe very well.
C. With all the blood thinners I was taking to avoid blood clots in my legs, and without hair on my head, I knew I would struggle mightily in the cold weather – which is the best time of year for duck hunting.
D. This was my son's first year at college; in fact, it was his first semester, and here we were talking about him skipping the next semester to go hunting with me.

It came down to this reality: It might just be my last duck hunting season alive. After much debate, we went for it. We lined up a hunting boat with a pull-up blind cover for my boy, and a big heater (and room for a hot thermos or two) for me. My wife and I scheduled a time to meet with his instructors, who agreed to let him skip a semester and hold a spot for him in the spring. They did advise – as did his mother and I - that this would put him way behind.

"Dad, if you're willing to do this for me, I will pay whatever price it takes to catch up," he said. "I will graduate with my class." His mind was made up!

So we hunted – right on through the pain and the chemotherapy treatments. We had a record take of waterfowl that season, and more importantly, we had some incredible heart-to-heart conversations in that duck boat. It was priceless. I felt confident that if I lost this battle with cancer, my boy was ready to handle not only his own affairs, but those of the family. What a great feeling of peace to know that love was stronger and tougher than any cancer could be.

He went back to school in the spring, and we still took every chance we could to be together. We'd watch some football, eat some dinner, and the next day go fishing with a chair for me at the water's edge. I would weep when he drove away. Under the captivity of cancer, every action seems to have such finality. When you don't know how much time remains, you don't take a moment of it for granted anymore.

During spring football drills as his team's athletic trainer, I found a way to be watching from the crowd. It wasn't easy. I'd been told to stay home and rest. I had chest tubes from my recent lung surgery dangling off of me, draining an unpleasant-looking fluid at seemingly the flow of a small creek. Not a good conversation-starter with the person sitting next to you. So I'd try to set up my chair next to a clump of bushes for some privacy, and I'd watch the drills. Still, I knew his graduation was a long ways off, and I was living on borrowed time.

It was another fine Christmas morning when I looked around at my family and thought I had everything I could ever want. That's when my daughter handed us a Christmas card with an ultrasound photo inside. Wow! We were looking at our newest grandchild.

Now I had another serious purpose. I had another birth and a graduation coming, and I was determined to be alive for both. Everyone get out of my way! I had the faith, the help and the mindset. *What cancer?*

On May 12, 2007, I watched with great pride as my son walked onto the stage to receive his hard-earned college diploma. I realized that he had worked as hard to stay in school during my illness as I'd worked to stay out of the hospital. I was now in what my oncologist called "no-man's land," since very, very few with my level of cancer make it this far.

I had another picture to put up on my mantle. This one told the story of a courageous young man who left for college, knowing that any day he could receive the call he feared the most. He knew how much I wanted him to get a college education; but what he didn't know was how bad I'd wanted to be there to see him complete it. We had both paid the price, and reaped the reward.

Hugging me in his cap and gown, he looked at me and said "Thanks, Dad, for being here."

I replied, "Thanks for giving me the goal."

22

Nine days later, miracle of miracles, I was alive to see new life enter the world again. Hoping that my cancer-weakened arms would hold him, I pulled my tiny second grandson, Carter, to my chest. His small warm body against mine brought healing to all the pain I had withstood. What a moment to remember. What a moment to cherish.

To witness my second grandson's birth and hold, kiss and hug that new life was overwhelming. How precious these moments are to a cancer patient. How much we need to live for tomorrow enough times to achieve our goal. Thank you, cancer, for making my family sacred again. Thank you "Carter Sauce" for extending your "Papa's" life.

ANOTHER CLOSE CALL

I had another brush with death in summer of 2007, and this one had nothing to do with cancer.

With all my goals accomplished to date, and more physical mobility with my illness than ever, I'd been working on some summer projects. The summer season is wonderful in North Idaho – great weather, beautiful lakes, biking trails and fishing. The fireworks show presented on the 4th of July by The Coeur d'Alene Resort is spectacular. It's become an all-day event for my family. We spend from 8 a.m. till midnight on the water, watching the grand fireworks display from our boat. With days like that, you could see how I could get distracted from my home projects. But I had "made up my mind" to get some things done with my newfound strength. One of those was a new deck for Sandi's flower garden.

My wife is a "flower freak." I mean that in the best of ways. Sandi loves fresh flowers in the house, around the house and especially on the deck. For Christmas one year I got her "Flowers for a Year," where she received a fresh beautiful bouquet of flowers every month (What a guy will do to go hunting!).

With our family growing, when the whole gang joined us for summers in North Idaho our existing deck filled up fast. I contacted Ken, "My 6 a.m., rock head contractor friend," to install a much-larger deck with a glass railing where Sandi could hang flower boxes. I'll admit she has a real gift. In her hands, that whole deck came alive with sights and smells, a "Garden of Sandi."

We all enjoyed the new deck that summer. I remember counting eighteen people on the deck, with furniture, grandkids, toys and the BBQ. My new deck seemed too small already!

That July morning, with family gone back home, I sat on the new deck enjoying my morning coffee and newspaper. The sun warmed my face as it rose above the tall pine trees for a new day.

As I swallowed my "little white pill," the T-100 Tarceva dose I needed daily, I thought back over the past four years. I was again overwhelmed by the fact that I was still alive and that I'd just spent a wonderful two weeks with my family. Cancer is bad, there is no doubt, I know! But the good that cancer has brought to me and my family is priceless.

After cancer, time together is never taken for granted. Each moment of every day is now more precious than the English language has words to express. I am blessed and I pray I will never allow the sacred to become mundane again.

From the deck, I looked around and noticed the intricate beauty of each flower along with their fragrant scents. They made me feel small in the whole picture of life. Humbled, I was content, and loved my place in it.

With the coffee gone, and the paper read, I turned to my morning project. After seeing Sandi drag a heavy hose around the house to water her new flower garden, I was going to mount a reel-up hose on the deck for her convenience. I made a quick trip to the hardware store, changed into my work clothes and grabbed my tool belt to install the reel. New hose in hand, I walked onto the deck for the connection.

All at once, the entire deck buckled beneath me, collapsing to the hard ground and taking me with it. BOOM! It felt and sounded like an explosion. I was trapped beneath the debris, and surrounded by shattered glass. I heard Sandi calling for me. Then she called 911, using her cell phone because the falling deck had knocked out power to our home.

I could hear the sirens coming. Sandi knelt beside me in the glass and flowers, praying through her tears. I prayed, too.

I had survived four major surgeries, four years of cancer and now a fallen deck. As I took stock of my surroundings, I felt something strange on my left side. I turned to look and was amazed to discover a metal sprinkler pipe, rising straight from the ground some 20 inches. The dagger was wedged perfectly between my chest and my left arm. I closed my eyes again to thank God for his divine intervention. I believe He landed me in the only place I could have fallen and still be alive to share this event with you. If I'd been just six inches to the left, that metal pipe would have severed my heart.

Sandi stared at me though eyes of fear and joy. We had just witnessed God's amazing grace in sparing me once again from the grip of death.

Just one week earlier, my entire family had been on this deck, with my 2 ½-year-old grandson Byron, "Mr. B.," following me everywhere. Thank God that today he was safely home with his mom. I am stubborn and hard-headed – that's my nature – but I know now that I have been set apart for something or maybe someone. Maybe you!

Whether you have six months to live or you clear it by six inches, if you have a pure vision of purpose and meaning for your life – which you must have to meet your challenge – death will have to take a number and wait in line. That's because the author of life is writing your book.

And there's still a lot of story left to tell.

Warrior Words

Hi Jim,

I saw Dr. Kelly today and she showed me all the scans of my brain and said the little spider cancer they worried about is gone and the rest looks great. They can't find any more bad guys. I go back to see her in six months. I will probably get three more chemos to make sure all the bad guys are gone and then an MRI. So it was a good day for me and a victory for my mentor. Add me to your list of successes. Thanks for covering my back and keeping me going with all the positive waves. I really appreciate it. You're a good guy for anyone to have on his side. Talk with you soon.

Feeling good today,
–Chuck

CHAPTER 2
Make Up Your Mind!

I once heard that you can tell the courage of a person by how much it takes to discourage them. I want you to know that if you have cancer, it can and will discourage you. But I also believe that you can develop an attitude that will overcome nearly anything. Take it from a guy who was given a death sentence – now eight years ago and counting!

I have seen the effects of cancer on myself and those I love. My mom, dad, father-in-law and grandfather are all gone because of this horrible disease. Since the day I was taken captive by cancer, many fellow warriors have died including my mentor, who you will soon meet in this book.

I spent countless hours with these people, trying to understand what was in their head and heart. The common bond was a will to survive, and survive they did, long enough to help others and make a life-changing impression on those around them. It might have been easier some days for them to simply give up. They might have saved themselves a lot of pain. To be honest with you, I had that conversation with myself, too, in my own darkest hours. But one of the things that cancer can't take captive – as long as you don't allow it to – is your mindset.

When I was 12, my mom became very ill with a rare life-threatening condition. My sister and I stayed with a family friend, while my dad made endless trips between his job and the hospital. One night, my dad was supposed to join us for dinner. I remember vividly how he came in the door screaming and crying. Running to keep up, I followed him into the bedroom and crawled up on the bed with him.

"Dad," I asked, "What's wrong? How's mom?"

"Son, your mom is dying and she may not make it through the night."

After some time and many tears, my dad got a call from the hospital that mom was doing better and not to worry about her that night.

Years later, I heard my mother's side of the same story.

"Oh Jimmy," she said. "I was in a dream and this brilliant light kept getting closer and closer. The heat from this light was intense but I had such a peace. I believe it was God wanting to ask me something. The light asked 'What can I do for you? What is the one thing you want most?'"

My mom, bless her unselfish heart, said, "May I see my children grow up? That's all I want." The light vanished, and in three weeks, she was home with us again.

From the day she came home, mom had a mindset to be committed to a course of action. Her illness took a lot out of her, but no matter what she had children to raise and the gates of hell would not stop her.

My mom died from colon cancer at the very young age of 56. But her mindset saw her children grow up, graduate and get married. She even met and spent precious time with four of her five grandchildren. My mom was living with us when she died. We would talk every day about life and how at peace she was. Her mindset carried her though some very bad times.

Her last words to me, holding my hand and praying with me, were these:

"Jimmy, you are a good man and you have been blessed with a wonderful helper and children. You fight to live for them with everything you've got."

Little did she know that I would need every bit of her determined mindset and more when I was diagnosed with terminal lung cancer myself at age 50.

On June 19, 2012, I celebrated my 59th birthday, thank God! It's very sobering to know that my mother died before this point in her life. When the word cancer came out of my doctor's mouth that day, I looked at my wife and children and the voice of my mom rang clear. The pain from her loss returned in a flash. I was determined that my own family must never feel this pain.

I've learned a lot about myself in the past eight years, both good and bad. Cancer has a way of holding up a mirror that shows you who you really are. I encourage you to take your own look, and decide if you like what you see.

I soon discovered that cancer was the loneliest experience I had ever had. It tried to isolate me into myself and drain my strength. Even with faith, family, friends and the great people at my cancer facility, I felt all alone. It felt like nobody understood.

That's why it's not enough just to see yourself in the mirror. You need more. On one hand, it's a very personal battle, where you alone must make up your mind to survive, to summon the strength from within. At the same time, you absolutely need others. I was lucky enough to have a mentor, and to have my faith, family, friends and the great people at my cancer facility.

My mom lived longer than anyone could have predicted. I believe it's because she lived for others and through them she gained her strength, not through herself. Cancer can and will take a lot from you. But I believe with the right mindset and attitude, you can live and enjoy what you have right now.

In many ways, it can be everything you ever dreamed.

Trust me, I know.

ONE DAY AT A TIME

Under the death sentence of cancer, my life became much more stable. Why? Because I quickly eliminated everything that was not relevant at the time. I became very focused on my only goal – to survive. To accomplish this goal, you can deal only with those things that will help you to live through that one day. That's what it takes.

You may say, Jim, I want a long life. I don't want to settle for just days. Well, my friend, you're lighting candles in the wind if you're not focused on day-by-day survival. You'll only reach the long term with the mindset to live for one more day. Survive today, and get your head ready to survive tomorrow. It might be the toughest thing you've ever done. Some days, I prayed to simply survive one more hour.

Your body is a marvelous piece of work that can withstand amazing brokenness. It is your mind that is the weakest link in the survival chain, and that is what you must make strong.

With cancer, there will be days when you won't want to make it. It's all right to feel that way – but don't stay there. Even on the worst days of chemo I refused to stay in bed. I got dressed and melted into my rocker for the day. My mindset was to not let cancer take me out. I have said many times that cancer might still kill me, but I will not be lying down when and if that time comes.

During some very intense chemotherapy I never missed a birthday party or celebration for anything or anybody. Sometimes I was so sick that lifting a fork to my mouth was an unbelievable task, yet I still managed to survive that day.

My oncologist is a great doctor. He's been on the cutting edge for me from the day we met. He always tells me, "You do all the work." What can this brilliant man do to help me in my head? You will find how lonely cancer is. Your family, bless their hearts, really doesn't understand that you and you alone have to fight – and some days they will not like the way you're acting. Tough! I have made up my mind to win this battle and if you don't like my game face on then don't look. But I can't allow compromise.

To fight something when you're healthy, as I was my entire life, is a matter of taking time and medicine to get better. I've never had a broken bone. Before I started my own business I worked for a company that offered sick leave. When I decided to leave I had six months of sick leave to use up.

Cancer is not like that. I will never be as physical as I was before cancer. It takes a toll on your body. The hardest part for me was suffering through all the pain of chemotherapy and its collateral damage just to have my blood marker go up again. Cancer takes a lot of work to defeat. And whether it's active or not, your cancer will be with you for the rest of your life. You will learn to live as a cancer patient without your physical strength. But our new strength of mind will help us face absolutely anything, even a reoccurrence of cancer.

REBEL OR REJOICE?

When you first hear you have cancer, you will have a wave of emotions come over you: faith, fear, anger, peace. Heaven or Hell. I can tell you I did! All these feelings can be destructive or constructive, fatal or life giving. You can give in or you can get creative.

I don't deserve cancer, I screamed inwardly. *I always considered myself a pretty good guy, husband and dad. I never smoked. It's not fair. Why me?*

But anger is not going to help you. I was mad as hell when the basement in my house flooded and ruined everything. Did it repair the basement? Will your "woe is me" heal you? Will you survive on anger alone? I don't think so.

You can and should rebel against cancer, but in a positive way. Instead of anger, seek peace; instead of rebellion, rejoice. You have been granted a new start on life. From this point on, you can renew your thinking and focus on what really matters: God, family and life. Even if you have screwed your life or family into a dysfunctional circus, cancer can be used to fix it. I know!

I am inspired by Daniel's story of being taken captive and having to live in an ungodly country against his will. He accomplished what he made his mind up to do because he had a clear purpose in life. Do you? I do now, thanks to cancer clearing my vision.

Maybe with cancer, for the first time in your life, you're faced with something you can't lie, steal, cheat or bull your way out of. That's what cancer did to me. I realized I was helpless, powerless and if I did not react to this new crisis in a positive way, I would also be dead.

The day of my cancer diagnosis, I resolved to make up my mind. I committed to a course of action. I determined to do what is right and not give in to the pressure or opinions around me. I resolved to be the man and the example God intended me to be.

I knew I would need time to repair a lot of brokenness, and the biggest part of the broken puzzle was me. With a potential six months to a year to live, that wasn't much time to fix fifty years of stuff. But I made up my mind to live through this – to repair and rebuild no matter what it took.

However many months of chemo it took – I made up my mind. However sick I got or how much hair I lost – I made up my mind. However many times a day I threw up, tried to eat, and threw up again – I made up my mind. However much pain I had after the lung surgery to remove the tumor, however much I hated walking around the hospital with chest tubes dangling, however many nights I woke up with a pool of water from the night sweats – I MADE UP MY MIND.

My prayer for you is this: Use cancer against itself. Use it to heal your angry and resentful heart. God still loved Daniel even though he allowed him to suffer much. God caused great things to happen in Daniel's life because he made up his mind to do the right things at the right time. God still loves you too. Use this time in your life – not to rebel any longer, but instead, to rejoice in that fact.

I encourage you to use this time to rebuild bridges that you have destroyed along the path of life. Call your ex-wife or ex-husband and talk to them about real life. Mend and renew your relationship with your children, if your will is to survive. Renew your love for your spouse who, like it or not, makes you a better person. Pass this new mindset on to your business, church, friends and any other cancer patient you can find.

I thank God for allowing cancer to change me into a better everything. I'll bet the cancer demons are mad but that's what can happen with faith, determination and the right mindset.

NOW YOU'VE GOT TO MAKE IT

There are days when the cancer war is so overwhelming that you want to give in, give up and raise the white flag. Every day is a new challenge. Even when the cancer is in remission, the war is still raging inside and out. Yes, I'm much stronger and able to enjoy more, but at the same time, since I'm not 100 percent in attack mode, I find my mind drifting.

It's our nature to forget pain, and forget bad things, only to allow ourselves to become consumed again with a non-purpose life. This culture in which we live does its best to destroy you and your thinking. It's so easy to be swept away again into this tidal wave of crap we call life.

I must remember the pain of chemo, the aching bones in my body after a blood-building treatment, the taste of metal mouth and the constant ringing in my ears. One look in the mirror at the marks left by chest tubes and lung surgery brings me back to reality. I hope you never suffer any of that.

Don't take for granted what you have accomplished during your war with cancer. If you have made it through one hour or eight years, be thankful for the life that God has given you. Nobody and nothing else gives life. In Daniel chapter 5, it tells me that God holds my life's breath in his hands and controls my destiny. Don't allow yourself to forget how precious life is.

Life becomes real when faced with death. Not some stupid reality show, but real life. Precious life that does not exist for things, glory, money or looks.

For the first two years with cancer, my life revolved around my La-Z-Boy chair, where I lived, ate, slept and spent nearly every waking moment. With severe deep vein thrombosis in both legs, I needed to keep my feet up. In front of that chair, my sweet wife posted every picture we had of family, daughter, her wedding, grandchild, hunting and fishing with my son. Some days the only reason I made it through was those pictures. My ultimate purpose was to live for them, not me.

I challenge you: Resolve to make up your mind. You must be able to face the serious issues head on. Find a way – when there is none – to survive. Search your heart and let it talk to you, and the things that are missing can be found. Knock and the door shall be opened.

Don't give up just because you have been taken captive. Remember that the faith of a very small mustard seed will do anything. Find a way to survive and you will cherish the change that cancer can make in your life.

Warrior Words

Cancer is a very lonely disease. While family and friends are supportive and sympathetic, usually they have no reference to what an individual with advanced cancer, or any cancer, is going to face in the treatment phase. Even your oncologist, who certainly has witnessed his or her patients' reactions to treatment, has not experienced, firsthand, the side effects of cancer treatment.

I met Jim Morrison shortly after March 2009, when I was diagnosed with stage 4 lung cancer. My oncologist at the time had suggested I get my personal affairs in order, since the advanced stage of my cancer would likely take my life within the next six months.

I learned of Jim Morrison's journey and that he had been diagnosed with stage 4 lung cancer and had survived, at that time, for nearly five years. He became my rock in helping me to understand the journey I would face. As is often said about cancer, the treatment can be worse than the disease.

In addition to being my mentor, Jim has become a dear and trusted friend. We talk and meet regularly to discuss this unusual journey we are experiencing.

–Jim Elder

CHAPTER 3
Don't Set Yourself Up

There I was, still in shock and denial of my oncologist's report. I tried to sort out every feeling, and most of all, I felt fear. I needed to sleep but it was the last thing I could do. I kept turning the pages of the Book of Daniel. I soaked up every word.

When I reached chapter 5, I read five words that made me sit straight up in my ICU bed: "You have set yourself up."

A profound realization hit me. All my life, I'd watched some of those closest to me pierce their own hearts with self-made grief. Worse yet, I'd turned around and done the very same thing.

Long before I was taken captive by cancer; in fact, from the day I was born, I had "set myself up" to become entangled in some pretty ugly messes. How about you? Let me ask you this: Do you know what to do when you find yourself in a hole? Stop digging! I learned the hard way that a shovel has two functions, to dig a hole or to fill it up. I've found that they are much easier to dig than they are to fill sometimes.

With cancer, I suggest you don't dig any new holes. Instead, use your bout with cancer as a shovel, and use it to start filling all the ones you've already dug.

DON'T PANIC

I had an onslaught of emotions when I was told I might have six months to live. I was angry, depressed, devastated, helpless, powerless and totally drained to empty. But I never gave in to panic. I urge you to do the same.

Everyone can experience different symptoms and side effects. The side effect you found on the internet that you fear the most? You may not even have it and never will. But you spent valuable energy, which you will always need to conserve, worrying about it.

I believe you are too vulnerable to read and look at everything out there. For the cancer patient, the war becomes more escalated if you're going to outlive this thing. You will become more desperate to find help. Be careful where you look and who you listen too.

I love my only sister but we are wired differently. Sometimes she drives me nuts. In 2009, she had been feeling ill for some time. I finally talked her into seeing a doctor instead of guessing and worrying about every disease out there. I told her to find what's wrong, get help and move on with life. She was a nervous wreck while she waited for the test results.

One night she called me in a panic.

"I might have signs of hepatitis," she said.

She rambled on and on about what type, what the side effects were, and how it would be treated. She was worried about missing work. She was terrified.

"How will I ever make it?" she said tearfully. "Oh Jim, I hate shots. Who will take care of my cats? I'm all alone. There's no way I can do it all."

Wait a minute, I thought. How did she know all this about a disease she hadn't even been diagnosed with?

"Sis, shut up a minute," I said, finally getting a word in. "I'll make you a deal. I'll trade whatever you think you have for my stage 4 lung cancer." It was like water off a duck's back – she just kept on hysterically. She finally ran out of air and I jumped in.

"Who have you been talking to?" I asked.

"Oh, nobody," my sister said. "On my way home I stopped and bought a book on the *ABCs of Hep*."

And you can guess the rest of the story. When she went in for her final test results, the doctor gave her a clean bill of health.

She had lost a week of sleep and spent a ton of emotional energy by filling her head with things she did not need to know. Just like her, I've met people who didn't even know yet what stage or type of cancer they had. All they knew for sure is that they had cancer – and by what they had seen and read online, they'd better pick their coffin color. They were already running and nothing was chasing them. DON'T PANIC!

By the way, I read a Book, too, and it tells me about my future. The difference is that I personally know, trust and have faith in the Author.

RELY ON WHAT YOU KNOW YOU CAN TRUST

There are three things I put my trust in: My faith, my family and my cancer facilities. Of course you have to do your part, but knowing you have these at your back makes a huge difference. In my opinion, if you don't have these, or if you have doubt about them, you should handle it now.

Most cancer facilities have support groups, and you should use them if you need to. I have even encouraged fellow cancer warriors to switch oncologists if they don't trust their skills. Most doctors are on your side, and they will do everything they have been trained to do. God bless the cancer professionals who work hard every day to save our lives. The rest is where your faith and family come in.

I realize that not everyone has a close-knit family. Or in this day and age, with many blended families, you may not really know someone to sink all your deepest emotions into. If you don't have immediate family, you will in the cancer ward. You will spend more time with them than with your own family. They are looking for support, too, and the sense of fellowship is strong in our little community. All cancer patients I've met have been great (with one notable exception) and very willing to share their war stories, both good and bad, with me.

Okay, now you can trust your family and your cancer center, but what about your faith?

I saved this for last because without a doubt in my mind, faith is the most important of the three. I have shared that my faith is in the Lord Jesus Christ. If you want political correctness, you're reading the wrong book. I'm certain that He extended my life because I have faith in the One who is helping me write this book eight years after He redeemed me from the chains of terminal lung cancer.

I will accept who or whatever you have your faith in, but I just pray it's right. I know better than to "set myself up" because this world says it's okay, or that all roads lead to the same place, or hey, you can be your own god, align your stars and all things are possible. Let me share a little secret with you: My faith is hard to live out faithfully, because it's being sure of what I hope for and certain of what I do not see. I realize not everyone has faith. It's your choice. My future with cancer has always been based on my faith. I was blind, but now I see.

DON'T SET YOURSELF UP

I don't understand it all, but I place every day of my life on someone I can't touch. Yet without any doubt I know He's real. If cancer kills me, does that mean my faith was a hoax? This unseen Person I write about and talk to every day, is He just in my head?

During my first year of bearing the cross of cancer, I was struggling with these questions. Early one morning, unable to sleep from the cancer-fighting drugs in my system, I was thinking about my cancer. It dawned on me that cancer is like faith. Bear with me here! In my case, I can't see the tumor in my lung, except by a CT scan.

I got to thinking about my invisible foe, and although I can't see it with my physical eyes, oh baby I know without doubt it's there. How? Because of it's effects on me. Like the wind – can you see the wind? Or do you see its results as the tree sways? When you turn your radio on, do you see the voice in the air coming to your antenna? Of course not, but without one doubt in your mind by turning the knob you are trusting something you can't see to be there for you.

I can't see who my faith is in, but the closer I get to his cross the more I can feel his effect. *And if cancer does kill me?* I will be at peace, knowing what I could not see I now can. Faith, family, friends and facilities are a powerful combination that you will need to beat cancer and survive one day at a time. I pray you can learn to trust in all four.

SEEK TRUTH AND STRENGTH

There are many ways to get information in the world today. It's smart to be up-to-date. Please understand that I am not against gathering all the information you can get your hands on. You do not want to be ignorant about what has you captive. I felt truth alone could help so that's what I was seeking. Since day one of my war on cancer, I've taken a list of questions with me to every checkup. I carry this piece of paper in my wallet so that when I think of something, feel something or someone questions something I think I should know, I write it down. I go over my questions with my doctor.

I have confidence in my doctor. I respect his knowledge and heed his advice. I don't need to research everything on my own. As a cancer patient, I always have questions, but I believe any information I obtain should be only to supplement the information my oncologist gives me.

Your doctor knows you better than anyone else – and they know what to say and when to say it. Trust him or her. Have questions? You should and will. Seek the correct answers from the best sources and avoid those that can "set you up" for unrealistic expectations.

I am encouraged when I read articles about new chemotherapy treatments that are being used now. I may need it someday. I love reading survivor stories. I receive a nationally published cancer magazine that is loaded with great information for the cancer patient. I greatly encourage you to seek the right knowledge about your condition, and I also urge you not to give in to doubting and loss of hope.

Along with seeking truth, seek strength. Cancer gave me something I was not used to having… time. I had time to just sit or lie down and think about things past, present and future. Yes, I had lots and lots of down time – it comes with the disease. You will use it to "set yourself up" or fill some old deep holes.

With a business, job, children and family in this fast-paced world we live in, how much time do you have every day to just sit and think? You can do this for hours, days, and even years with cancer. No time limits and boundless hours of sitting and thinking. I found by looking back into my past I would gain renewed strength for the future.   As I once heard, "Your future may be in your past."

I found strength through things I survived that devastated me at the time. When my mom died with colon cancer, I really did not think at the time that I could live any longer without her. She was my rock of refuge when the seas of my dysfunctional family would rise. My dad was an alcoholic and he set both himself and his family up big time. I survived.

Because of his condition, I spent a lot of time instead with my mom's dad, who I nicknamed "Paw." An old-school Italian, he taught me more about life than I ever learned in school. My business ethics and public relations skills are based on what he taught me many years ago. Sorry, present day-wisdom, I will practice old-school common sense anytime. It's what I taught my kids, and now I am going to brainwash my grandchildren with it.

I was born and raised in San Diego, where my dad was stationed in the Navy. There, I first knew "Paw." He was a very hard-working man. As a full-blooded Italian he had a great camaraderie with all the tuna boat captains. Many times I was invited to board a boat and meet the crew.

Paw would start work at 11 p.m. and was done by 7 a.m. When he came home, he'd find me packed and ready to go fishing, and off we'd go to the Shelter Island Pier. I can still remember glancing over to see my Paw nodding off where he sat on his five-gallon bucket, tired from his all-nighter, but still willing to fish with his grandson. He was my first mentor. He never realized what a wonderful lesson he taught me: fishing was not about his needs, but about mine.

This is how I learned the word that spells love more than anything for kids – TIME. You are "setting yourself up" if all you give your kids is rushed love. Why? Because you know what they really want is your time.

When my Paw and fishing buddy passed away from lung cancer, I was absolutely crushed. I have missed him every day since, but I survived. My dad continued in his alcoholism, which caused huge problems between us in my early years. During his captivity to the bottle, when he had idle time he continued to dig holes for himself – holes that in the end he could never climb out of.

There was one terrible pit he dug that was so deep that he pulled me in with him. It wasn't alcohol, since I refused to drink with him. I guess he was starving for some kind of relationship with me, because he kept trying – even when I'd refuse. The only thing he never tried was time.

After I met my junior high school sweetheart – now my wife – we were inseparable. My dad thought it would be a good idea to show me a thing or two about the birds and the bees. He had at that time a very large collection of adult movies hidden away. When you're 15, bad time together with your dad is better than none at all. That day, I learned what captivity was all about.

Since that encounter, pornography became a tragic hole that I continued to dig, "setting myself up" for failure for years to come. I knew better! I saw what happened to my dad because of it, but I did it anyway.

I want you to know that my dad and I became friends again. Love is all that's left in a relationship after all the selfishness has been removed. While in his last rehabilitation facility, we dealt with all the hurt, bitterness and anger. The power of forgiveness is a wonderful thing to experience. At last, my dad gave me his time, which I spelled LOVE. He hugged me and said he loved me and that he was sorry. For six months, my dad and I rejoiced in our time together right up until the lung cancer took my new best friend from me.

I felt so cheated after he died. All that precious life and time wasted. I was burdened again with a broken heart because of cancer, but I survived!

It had been years since I'd reviewed these memories, both good and bad. Cancer gave me the time. I should be furious at cancer for taking the ones I loved so much. I could have easily "set myself up" by digging my thoughts into a hopeless pit. But instead of panicking, I put the cancer to good use.

With the inner strength from my past, I "made up my mind" that I could survive another bad event, my fight with cancer. I know

WHAT IF YOU ALREADY HAVE?

My counsel is that you don't "set yourself up" – but what if you already have? Can you make a comeback? You must! Just because I've made some bad choices and "set myself up" doesn't mean I'm going to be a doormat, welcome cancer in and let it have its way. Hell, no! I'm going twelve rounds with my opponent. Let Him who controls my destiny decide the champion.

You don't need cancer to use this great lesson. I know of many kinds of captivity that will destroy you and your family much quicker than cancer. And so do you.

My dad was a broken man at the end of his life. Not simply in a spiritual sense, although I believe that's also true. But also because he knew all along that his very bad choices would continue to lead to failure. I watched my alcoholic father lose his wife, children, home and business. And after all that, he still continued to dig. Remember, YOU alone must stop digging.

After watching my father's plunge, could I stop my own downfall? My own addiction to porn had become a very real problem. It was starting to affect my own wife, children, home and business. I realized that I was heading toward the same failures as my father, just using a different "drug of choice" to dig the hole.

One day, my princess daughter set up a family meeting. She called me at work and said, "You will be home at four o' clock today. We need to talk." After a brief discussion with our family, she pointed her finger straight at me and bluntly stated, "Dad, knock it off! Or get out of our lives. We will not tolerate it one day more."

This is a most unpleasant memory, and I entrust it to you simply to prove that you, too, can gain strength from the roughest times. I still remember the pain of that day, both mine and theirs. I had "set myself up," even when I knew better. But by the grace of the Lord whom I choose to serve, and by faith in His power and not my own,

He paid my ransom and I was released from my own self-dug prison on March 26, 2001.

Little did I know that years later I would be diagnosed with lung cancer. But now I took cancer on with a whole different attitude. Still having the rope burns around my neck from the last captivity, I decided from day one not to make bad choices and not to trust in myself, but in the God who can raise the dead.

Today, I'm fed up with what I call my Self-Induced Nonsense, or S.I.N. This was a very hard lesson to learn and live by, but oh how valuable. You have S.I.N. in your life too (also known as Self-Inflicted or Self-Indulgent Nonsense!). You can and will be forgiven if you choose to give it up and live the way you know is right. But it's not easy to give up something we are born with in our DNA.

We practice and perfect our S.I.N. until it destroys everything we are and all who are around us. Do you really want to be like everyone else? I don't! I want to be "set apart" for something, not conforming to this messed-up world. I want a renewed mind so I can understand what's really real and what's not. I was blind but now I see and understand.

Someday, you will have to confront your own S.I.N. If you're like me, you'll eventually ask yourself, "What did I ever gain from my S.I.N that I'm not ashamed of?" If this makes you aware that the real truth is available, you will find Him and He'll set you free. He certainly did for this sinner.

My prayer is that if you have cancer – or anything else that is holding you captive – that you seek this grace immediately. I love you, my fellow warrior.

WHY ME?

I am a blessed man. I have been given grace where none is deserved. I've been fortunate many times over – first to be still alive, and then to witness so many miracles of life around me.

With cancer, it's natural to ask "Why me? Why did I get this?"

Sometimes I find myself asking instead: "Why me to beat the odds? Why me to accomplish all these goals?

"Why me when so many die from cancer? Why me that I'm still here for my family? Why me to whom God would show favor? Why me who would live long enough to write this book?"

Well, why not?

To all who have been taken captive by cancer, or by anything, there's something I want you to know. Despite the worst of circumstances, faith, love and hope can endure. You will be amazed at what you can do when you have to. I would encourage you to look past your pain to see someone else's. Many years ago, a heroic young man named Jesus did just that, and he set the captives free – and me too.

SET APART FOR SOMETHING

Some people might see the figurative "C" on your forehead, and count you as doomed. Don't listen! How many times have you heard that cancer is a death sentence? Well, I believe you can't trust everything you hear. Remember how the world as we knew it was going to end in Y2K?

Now, serving the time I've been given to live, I believe we are here for a purpose. We may never see it or understand it, but be here we must until our work is completed. I want you to know you have been set apart for something important. There will be rough nights when you'd rather not wake up the next morning. Remember, someone in your life needs your strength. Stay alive, and accomplish your purpose.

Warrior Words

When I met Jim Morrison in 2009, I knew there was something special about him that would change people's lives. His story was a remarkable one of courage, strength and heartfelt compassion. He is one of those rare people who has descended into the depths of pain and despair and arose stronger and with a heart full of grace to share with others.

Jim had agreed to tell his story for the Kootenai Health Foundation's Festival of Trees, benefiting cancer services at Kootenai Cancer Center that year. His story and the manner in which he told it provided hope and a battle plan for others in similar circumstances. By setting goals to achieve at each stage of the journey, he was able to fight through the worst days of his life with the help of his family, faith, friends and as he calls it, facilities – the doctors, technology, medicine, and nurses who were his allies in the battle.

At that year's annual Festival Gala, Jim gave such an empowering speech that we quickly raised the money needed to establish a new program focusing on wellness at the Kootenai Cancer Center. He inspired the crowd, taking them with him on his journey and offering them hope that they, too, might help to change lives through their gifts. At the heart of his message, though, was the incredible love he had for his family. They were the focus of each goal that took him through the darkest days.

Jim touched me personally as well. Early in our conversations, a friend of mine was diagnosed with lung cancer. This vibrant, healthy individual who I admired and seemed to me to be the picture of wellness was facing a myriad of decisions and had to choose a path through this new challenge. I felt that I had been given the gift of knowing both of these wonderful men and their individual stories and that if I could connect them, something beyond anything I could offer might happen. Indeed, I asked Jim if he would be willing to allow me to offer his name and number to my friend and be open to a call if he so chose. They did connect and that friendship, I believe, was inspired.

Jim has used the lessons of his journey to help many along this difficult path. Those journeys clearly don't always lead to the same destination, but the people he helps certainly find understanding in a manner that no one else can offer who hasn't traveled that road.

I thank Jim for writing this book and thereby reaching out to help even more people facing the challenge of cancer. Jim and his wife, Sandi, and their family are all inspiring in their strength, courage, love and generosity in their desire to support others. I thank Jim and his family for joining all of us at the Kootenai Health Foundation in our journey to change lives. He makes us all better.

–Teri Farr, MPA, CFRE
 President, Kootenai Health Foundation

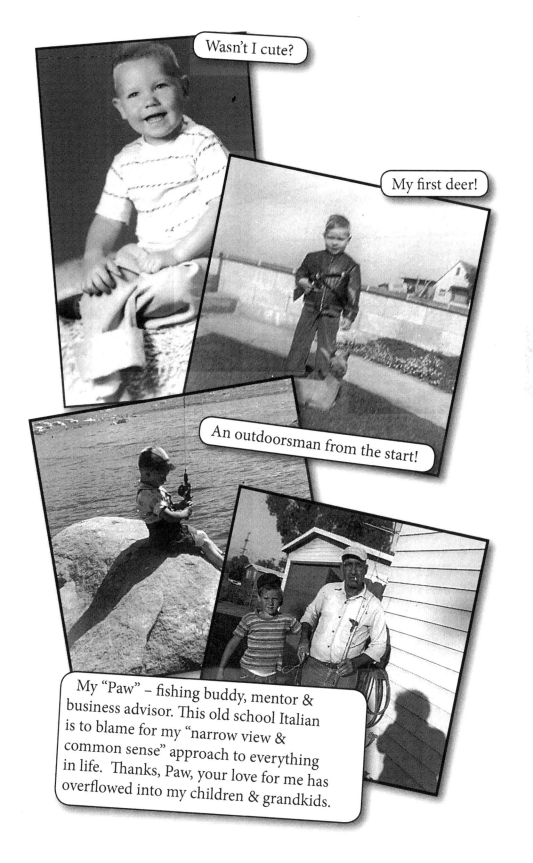

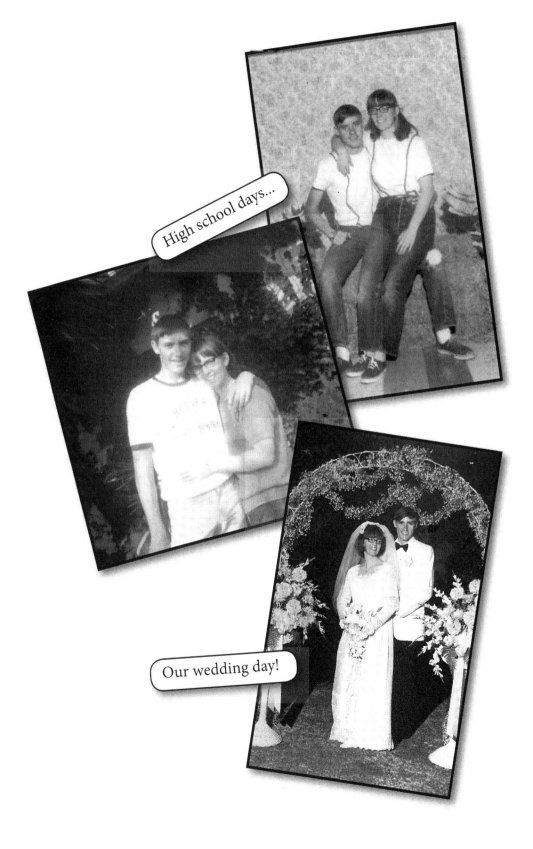

Our new home in Idaho...

Comfort Heating & Air

1st company truck

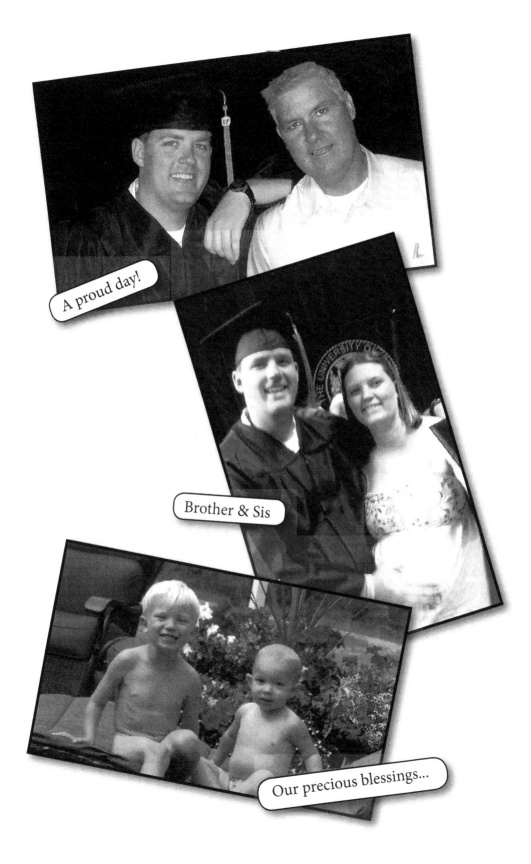

A proud day!

Brother & Sis

Our precious blessings...

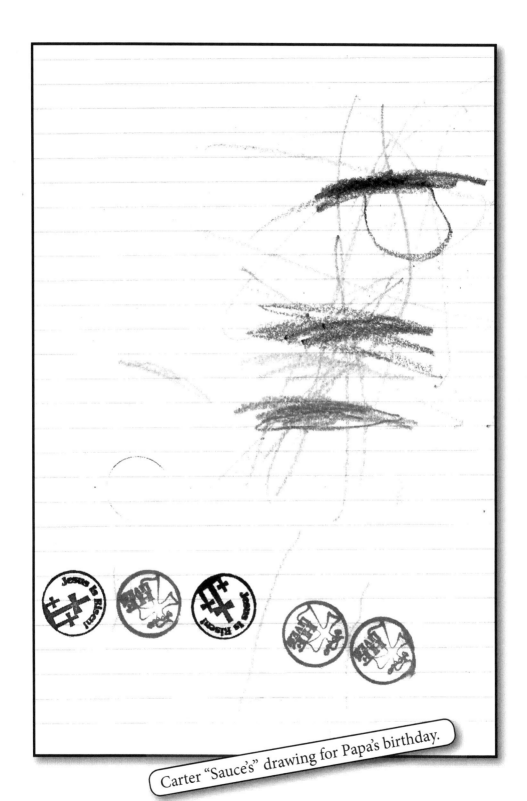

Carter "Sauce's" drawing for Papa's birthday.

CHAPTER 4

Cancer Has A Way of Humbling... Let It!

I'm not a guy who likes to wait for anything. Driven by a "Triple Type A" personality, I've spent my whole life in the fast lane. My brain worked better there and I made more money there. I also drove my family crazy there. Patience is not a virtue of mine. It slowed me down.

I remember hearing once, "There are three kinds of people: Those who make things happen, those who watch things happen, and those who wonder, 'What just happened?'" I will admit this trait of making things happen has taken me down some unfamiliar roads way too fast, only to find a dead end or two. The crashes can be big, but it also gave me more chances and increased my odds. After all, one of those roads might take me to the finish line. I always figured that one day at the age of, say 120 years old, I would finally slow down and be a bit more patient.

LANE CHANGE

And then came January 2004. I had just received my diagnosis. The word cancer, as it first echoed off the walls of my hospital room, continued to penetrate my ears and those of my loved ones. With weakened knees, aching hearts and lungs that were gasping for air, we were stopped in our tracks, as if our ticket on the train of life had expired. Our ride was over. We were to be escorted off and left in an abandoned ghost town with no hope.

Our lives were now slowed by waiting extra-long days for the biopsy report. The wait drove me crazy. Unfamiliar with the procedures of cancer treatment, I would say, "We're wasting time! Let's get going with the chemotherapy." Kym, my nurse daughter, in her loving, compassionate way, would tell me, "Knock it off, Dad!"

I was slowed to a crawl, not only from my gallbladder being removed, but also by the news that both of my lungs, along with the sac around my heart, were saturated in cancerous bloody fluid that required immediate attention. My "Triple Type A" was now weakly holding on to "Type Single D."

During my career in the heating and cooling business, I never let sickness slow me down. This cancer sickness, unlike anything I had ever experienced, held me completely bedridden for my two-week stay in the ICU. Who I thought I was – and what I thought I could accomplish – was completely out of my hands. My "make things happen" was now done by my team of doctors. All I could do was watch, and wonder "What just happened?"

I have to thank my excellent caregivers – including Dr. Antoine Sarkis, who we call 'my guardian angel', at the Kootenai Cancer Center for their patience with me. For the first time in my fifty years, I was slowed to a pace that I'd never experienced before. In fact, I was afraid to proceed too fast, fearing that they might find more bad news (if that's possible with stage 4 lung cancer!). As the days passed and I became weaker and weaker, it was apparent that cancer would have an effect on me. It was up to me to decide if that effect would be for the worse, or for the better.

In time, my condition stabilized. I felt very lucky to still be alive, since at one point only two hours had meant the difference between me being released from the hospital, or from its morgue. Now, I was preparing for the war ahead. My cancer center did a great job in covering all the bases – not just for me, but for my family, too. How valuable was my nurse daughter Kym? Priceless! She would "doctor talk" with my team of professionals, and then turn around and translate to me, as a simple heating guy, exactly what was going on.

My last procedure before chemotherapy was the surgery to install an infusion port. By the way, if you are going to receive long-term infusion treatments, consider this procedure. It is a must-have that will save you much pain and discomfort, and with cancer, we already have plenty of that. This simple procedure gives the medical staff one place to draw blood and inject the necessary drugs, instead of having to stick you constantly in many places.

With my left front shoulder still tender from my port, I was nervous, but ready for my first round of chemotherapy. Why my left shoulder? As crazy as it sounds, I was planning to hunt waterfowl that coming fall with my son, Jeff. I asked my doctor to put the port on the left side, because with it on the right side I couldn't have shot my gun. Cancer doesn't mean you're dead. It does, however, make you set a goal and slow down to smell the gunpowder.

THE NIGHT BEFORE THE CHAIR

It was one day before my first chemotherapy treatment. My body was weak, but my mind was still running strong. There was a real conflict between what I wanted to do – running my business – and what I knew I had to do if I wanted to survive. Once again, I realized that I would need a new mindset if I were going to beat cancer.

The word "cancer patient" was taking on new meaning. Everything about the disease had become a waiting game. And here I was, waiting for the dreaded "chair" where I would get my first chemotherapy infusion.

It was a long and scary night. The nervous fear alone made me so sick I couldn't sleep. I felt that the next day I would walk into a room and walk out changed forever, that I would never again have the health that God had so blessed me with. I didn't have a clue what the chemotherapy would do to me, but I had witnessed its effect on my loved ones.

In the early morning hours, my weird mind imagined a convicted murderer, waiting for the chair in which the death sentence would be carried out, counting each minute until life was no more. I imagined what it must be like to be escorted to that chair, and then feel the needle penetrate into my skin. I imagined the relief of the last-minute pardon that sometimes comes.

I knew that very morning I would be escorted to a chair. I would feel the needle penetrate into my port. With my junior high school sweetheart by my side, we would hold hands with a new grip, one in which I would feel her pain for me. *I didn't want this! These were circumstances that I did not create! I am not guilty!*

And yet, I must go. I need what could be this lifesaving infusion, created by man, although engineered by the author of life Himself. *If man has the authority to pardon man, and extend life, then how much more authority does He who was raised from the dead have to extend the life of whom he chooses?*

THE WAITING ROOM, NO WAY!

My very nervous wife and I entered the elevator, hesitant to push the 2nd floor button to the cancer ward. I was thinking that if I had only one choice from every person alive today, only my best friend could help me through this ordeal. I met her while I sweated over a 9th grade spelling test that would secure my position on the track team. Today, again willing to help, she is at my side encouraging me to survive cancer.

As the bell tolled and the double door slid open, we took a short walk hand-in-hand down the lonely hall. As my other hand paused on the cancer treatment ward doorknob, both Sandi and I took one last gulp of fear.

What I hadn't envisioned during my night terrors was the time-consuming paperwork and instructions. "Mr. and Mrs. Morrison, please have a seat. We will be right with you." *Are you kidding me? It's like calling time out to "ice" the kicker before an attempted field goal!* Trying to find a hunting magazine to distract my mind, I realized why there was a puzzle table set up in the corner. We waited restlessly.

That vision of the death chair still fresh in my mind, I looked around the waiting room at the others. *Do they feel what I feel?* All of these warriors, both men and women, were waiting for cancer treatments of some kind. Some had helpers by their side while others were alone. All were in the battle for their life. All had been taken captive by cancer, and I knew that neither the patient nor the helper were immune from the mind games that come with it.

I didn't see statistics; I saw people who were full of fear and hoping against very bad odds that they would still be alive for their next birthday. These were real people in the most authentic "reality game" ever played. *Cancer is not a game you play for money and hollow fame. This is not the crap our televisions try to brainwash us with. This is real reality!* The prize that's awarded to those who finish with a breath is real life. And for the warriors who fight hard, but for reasons we may never know do not get that gift of life, the consolation prize is a very real peace from that war.

What if I could give everyone in this cancer ward right now a choice between fame and fortune versus life itself? What if they could have endless money and worldwide fame, weighed against freedom from cancer and many happy birthdays to come? What would everyone, without a doubt, choose?

My mind ran full bore with these thoughts while I waited for "the chair." I realized that cancer is no respecter of persons, and as a patient here, neither was I. Here, I could care less about your looks, your political preference or even what religion you follow. Here in the "cancer ward," I was with real life "American Idols," men and women who had forged a path through the jungle of cancer, who were willing to welcome me to the war, to accept me just as I was and help me to pick up the trail.

In the cancer ward, we are all warriors marching in sync and fighting for the grand prize of precious life. Some win, others die, but either way we have been singled out to play the ultimate reality game. *I choose VICTORY! How about you?*

THE INFUSION ROOM

Finally! We were greeted by a very friendly nurse, "Mr. and Mrs. Morrison, hi! My name is Peggy." As she led us into the infusion area, I told her that my daughter was a nurse, and that Kym would also love the frog designs on her colorful smock.

As we walked past others receiving their treatments, I realized that *I hated cancer.*

I tried to share an encouraging smile or a nod of my head. I knew I'd be spending a lot of time here, so I was trying to make a friendly impression – without relaying the absolute fear that had now taken over my body from the inside out. Some people responded kindly, many were in no kind of mood for acknowledgment, and others didn't even realize we had walked by.

Another nurse dressed in full hazmat-type attire excused herself to pass. *What kind of place is this, where nurses must wear protective clothing so they don't expose themselves to the poison they are infusing into my fellow warriors?*

Sandi's grip on my hand was now cutting blood flow off to my fingers.

"Mr. Morrison, please have a seat."

I couldn't do it. I was freaked out beyond belief by a simple chair. I felt all eyes were on me. I was guessing that everyone here was this nervous on their first visit.

"Jim, I'm here to help you. It will be all right," Peggy said softly.

As I slowly turned to take that seat, I recognized someone across the room, a former business colleague named Brian. I asked for a moment's respite from the chair and went over to him.

"Brian, what in the world? I can't believe it."

"Jim," he said. "Why are you here, visiting someone?"

"No sir, I have cancer! Today is my first session."

"Oh my," he said. "What are the chances of us meeting in an infusion room?"

I said, "Brian, I will be here for some time from today forward. I hope we can talk again soon. Have the best day you can, and by the way, thanks again for understanding my situation years ago."

Still amazed at seeing this guy, I returned again to the dreaded chair, uncomfortable but ready. Peggy, now wearing her own hazmat uniform, began my first session of chemotherapy. As I had imagined, I felt the prick from the needle penetrating into my skin. From the tears in Sandi's eyes, she felt that pain too.

Now we had to settle in for a long five-hour treatment. It was clear that I would have to deal with my restless spirit. By now I was quite aware that the road to remission would only be achieved in the slow lane.

I was not in control here, in fact, there was no doubt the cancer held me captive. But the way I saw it, captivity couldn't kill me. *Fear and faith are opposites. You can feel both, but you can only act on one.*

DAYS OF OUR LIVES – IN THE INFUSION ROOM

The first two hours passed quickly. I couldn't stop talking about what a coincidence it was to see Brian there. When I thought back to my insights from the book of Daniel, I realized once again that God is in total control of all things. Way back when I started my own heating and cooling company, Brian had been the service manager of another company that would not agree to pay me what I asked. Fortunately, we'd never been at odds, and we had even referred jobs to each other. Over the years it was rare to run into him. The last little chat we'd had was at a wholesalers' Christmas party, where he congratulated me for doing exactly what I told him I would do. Now twelve years later, we were fellow cancer warriors.

Relaxed enough now, or maybe just exhausted, with Sandi on guard at my side and in Peggy's skillful hands, I fell into a deep nap in my chair. I woke in disbelief to hear what was happening in the curtained area next to us.

A young man was going ballistic, yelling at the top of his cancer-filled lungs.

"I don't have time for this!" he screamed out. "I have a business to run. My wife is *(blankety blank)* useless! She knows nothing about my business. Without me this whole thing is gone. I want the *(blankety blanking)* doctor here now, get this *(blankety)* treatment done and it better be quick! I have more important things to do than waste my time here with you clowns."

How's that for setting yourself up?

Now I was already not in the best of moods, knowing I was about to bend my knees against my will at the altar of cancer. I hated the fact that I would have to allow poison to fill my body. I wanted to get out of my chair, pull the curtain aside, and meet the guy face to face. I wanted to look into his lifeless eyes and bury him alive.

"Knock it off you arrogant (blank)!" I wanted to say. "You have the right to remain silent. Use it! Most of us in this room want to live and enjoy life. If you trust in your pride-filled self so much, what are you doing here? Go home and heal yourself. These "clowns" are trying to save your selfish, prideful existence."

My wife gave me that look I have learned over the years not to cross. Reluctantly, I obeyed and kept my mouth shut. Still, I wanted to look at him, just to see if pride was as ugly as it sounded. *I'm just a former heating guy, not a doctor, but I know this: "Pride goes before destruction, and a haughty spirit before a fall." Pride will never heal you.*

CANCER HAS A WAY OF HUMBLING – LET IT

I never heard that young man again, even though I was in and out of that infusion room for the next three years. I believe that moment in time was by Divine intervention. I needed that lesson. I was very much struggling myself that day. I had other things I wanted to be doing, too.

It brought to mind the words I had read that early January morning in the ICU, "And those who walk in pride He is able to humble." (Daniel 4:37) Being made humble will either adjust your attitude so you can become a better person, or unravel your false sense of control. For us self-made men and women, that's a tough pill to swallow.

Pride can never heal or make you better, but it can without fail destroy you. Pride and cancer together have only one goal – destroy and kill. You can beat them both! But you will need help. Have you ever asked for help before? Do you know how? Have you ever allowed someone else to help you? Or does that just seem like a sign of weakness?

I wonder sometimes about that angry young man in the infusion room. I wonder if he ever asked for help. I wonder if he lived or died.

I never wanted cancer. I still don't. But I know that pride will not win me the war against cancer or any other captivity. I know I can't do it alone. Your bout with cancer may be your wakeup call. Don't let your pride keep you from asking someone to help answer it for you. He is able to humble those who walk in pride. I know this is true because He humbled me big time.

After I was diagnosed with deep vein thrombosis, my doctor made urgent plans to install a blood clot restraining device. He also insisted that I walk immediately. I would complain about how much my legs hurt, walk a short distance, and start moaning again. My wife, as well as the medical staff, was willing to help me walk but I wanted to do it on my own. They suggested I use a walker, but I refused.

That night, I heard a helicopter land on the roof of my hospital. That sound usually meant that a life-or-death situation was underway. There was a lot of action on my floor of the ICU that night. When my doctor made his rounds the next morning, I asked him what had happened.

"Someone was involved in a motorcycle accident," he said. "His injuries were life-threatening. They airlifted him here, and that's all I can say."

Before my doctor left he asked me "Are you walking?"

"Yes," I said. "But it's very uncomfortable. Both legs just ache."

"Are you having someone help you as you walk?"

"No, I don't need help," I said stubbornly.

In a very nice way, that doctor told me, "Tough. Walk!"

So I began to walk. On my daily shuffle around my floor, I passed the room where the motorcycle patient was lying still. A couple days later, he was awake, and I introduced myself as his neighbor. "Thank you for stopping," he said.

I stopped again the next day, eager to talk to him. He was sitting on the edge of his bed this time, and I was blown away by what I saw.

He had no legs. That night I'd been busy complaining about the pain in my legs, the doctors had been busy cutting off both of his to save his life.

I've never been so humbled as I was by this polite 20-year-old who had suddenly found himself without legs. I realized right then that my pride would not help or heal me.

Who was I to complain about my legs when this young man had none? He is able to humble and I am a blessed man because I allowed him to humble me.

I continued my walks with renewed vigor. I must admit that it was a lot easier now that I asked my wife to help me. The staff even took turns. They said it was "fun to help." The walks gave me time to really get to know them, something pride would never have allowed.

Today, my journey with cancer is built on faith, not on pride. I'm convinced that you will not start to heal completely until you're real with your pride. The cancer may not kill you, but your denial of pride will destroy you. I pray for people whether they are full of cancer, pride or both. I know which one is worse. I would rather have cancer take me fast while in peace with my God, myself and those around me, than to be actively destroying myself and everything around me as I commit slow-motion suicide with pride.

AN UGLY VIEW IN A BEAUTIFUL PLACE

I don't like to tell this next story, but I think you should hear it, anyway.

A friend called me to say that a mutual acquaintance of ours had just received a very bad biopsy report. He didn't have much time to live, and he and his family were in shock. My friend suggested I call, thinking maybe I could be of help to someone who was newly diagnosed and scared to death.

It's awkward at best, making the call to someone I have known, and now is a fellow cancer patient. He recognized my name, was cordial, and invited me to meet him at his house the next afternoon.

On my way there, I pulled to the side of the road and prayed. He needed help and so did I.

His very attractive wife opened the door, and along with their children, invited me inside their majestic custom home. The man came into the room and quickly led me outside onto the deck. We had a short but very intense talk, and agreed that I would return to see him as we began this journey together.

But as time went on things started to change.

I drove to see him twice a month or so. It was a beautiful drive. The road wound along the lake and climbed up though the pine and fir trees. Rounding the last turn, it was postcard perfect. The whole mountaintop opened up and you could see for miles. I once had to stop to allow a mother black bear to escort her twin cubs to their favorite meadow.

On summer evenings, surrounded by mountains in every direction, we would sit and talk on the open deck of his huge log home. When the sun sank over the lake for the evening, it was just too beautiful to put into words.

After a few visits, I noticed that the family was not allowed to be around. Other than hello and goodbye, I had no communication with his wife or children. Also, I felt he was uneasy talking about dying. This bugged me, since at this time death was fresh on my mind. I was into my cancer two years and battling daily.

This man was a very powerful public speaker with a worldwide reputation. It meant nothing to me, but I could tell that it did to him. I saw that he was in captivity, but I wasn't sure if cancer was his captor. What was he really fighting against?

As you know by now, the Book of Daniel is my handbook. After returning home one night from another frustrating visit, I rocked my "Old Faithful" La-Z-Boy back to get my legs up and read Daniel chapter 4. Wow! I was struck with a clear insight about what was happening with the family I'd been struggling to help.

Sandi, who had also spent some time with the man and his family, confirmed exactly what I'd realized, saying, "He is a control freak who is too proud to have cancer." Wow!

Positive now that pride was the real source of his captivity, I felt that I must tell this family the truth. I knew how my own past pride had blinded my eyes and stole my dreams. If there was going to be a victory here, it had to be addressed.

On my next visit to their mansion on the mountaintop, I was loaded for bear, not for the mama and her cubs, but to make or break a relationship. Could I, with help from He who can humble, open this man's pride-blinded eyes to see how he was setting himself and his family up for total destruction? Would he accept help or die controlling his situation on his own? Would he continue to divide and separate or would he drop the sham, let the dust clear and allow love and humility to heal him and his broken family?

With my "Daniel handbook" in my briefcase, in I went for our afternoon visit. A half-hour into our discussion, the ship hit the iceberg and began sinking rapidly. Was it something I said? Suddenly his wall was up and thick and I was not allowed to look over. After a very quick prayer in his office with him, I sprinted through the kitchen where his family was quarantined until I left.

With my final thank you and goodbye, I was hurried out and on my way down the not-so-beautiful-anymore drive. Before entering the highway I prayed for him, his family and myself for wisdom to handle this ticking bomb...

It was only a few months later that I was attending that man's funeral, hugging his beautiful widow in the foyer of their church before his funeral service. I gave each of his children a pat on the head. Looking at what was left of this family broke my heart.

I knew he'd had a chance to beat that cancer. But pride is gasoline on the fire.

The funeral was strange, cold and calculated. His family sat on one side, and her family on the other. The room was thick with tension.

When the service began, our mouths hung open with amazement when the man's face and voice came onto the projector screen in a videotaped message. Even in parting, he had pre-recorded and controlled his own funeral service. He had taped a prideful tribute to himself and an angry diatribe against others, and insisted that it be played.

It seemed that this poor 43-year-old man had lived in his own darkness for so long he could not face the light. Not being able to control cancer himself was overwhelming. His pride would not allow others to see his pain and struggle. Instead he blamed anything and everyone within range. He was at war in his own body, trapped deep in a hole he had dug.

The big screen made him look bigger than life, which is what he thought of himself. He carefully controlled the whole service from his coffin. He took his final shots at family and friends and God. The belittling of his wife, her family and God, railing against them in blame for his death, was unbelievable and so full of pride it made me sick.

When I looked for his wife after the service, my friend told me that when the recorded message started, she had taken the children and left. Now she was finally free from his pride and able to start a new life.

And here's the craziest part of this story. I've told you how devastating pride can be. I've told you how those who walk in pride are made humble. But how do you explain this?

Remember, the man with the strange, selfish funeral had made his money as a world-renowned speaker with a strong voice.

Tell me this – with all the various forms of cancer that can attack the human body... *Why did he die of throat cancer?*

PRIDE IS YOUR ENEMY

About four years before I was diagnosed with lung cancer, I met this guy named Ken in a small church group who had all the same problems that I was facing. Both of our families were on the brink of destruction due to our actions. We both owned our own businesses, but we didn't know how much longer we could survive. Our neat little worlds were crumbling around us, but why?

We went to coffee together. What we planned as an hour-long talk went three hours. Like two boxers, we were feeling each other out, getting into each other's head, feeling standoffish at best. We blamed everything wrong in our worlds on everyone but ourselves.

I really liked this guy. It was like looking into a mirror – we both knew everything about anything and everybody. We both were self-made, bold but hollow, very strong yet so fragile. We were both real "men's men," yet we lived behind a wall of self-doubt and the fear of failure.

We learned that both of us had previously tried to break over the top, only to be talked down or knocked down by someone else, usually someone who should have been building us up instead. Our trust in others had been destroyed so many times that we now allowed no one to penetrate our wall. *And if you cherish your face? Don't try looking over that wall!*

We never spoke the word pride in three hours, and yet it was the sole source of our problems. I think we knew it in our hearts. And I think we were prepared for the destruction that was stalking so very close behind just waiting to devour.

MY NEW "ROCK HEAD" FRIEND

Over time Ken and I became very good friends – really, more like brothers. It was one of those times in my life that now remind me what the Book of Daniel says, "He holds my life breath in his hands and controls my destiny." (Daniel 5:23) Please remember, at this time I didn't even know that Daniel had a book!

After hours of talking, we realized that we were both selfish, blind "rock heads" who were full of pride and needed to shape up. It was a long, painful process but we both survived, and more importantly, so did our families.

It was another good lesson: Let your wall down just enough to see who's on the other side. They might want to help. They might just understand more than you bargained for.

When I was in the ICU and needed help? My "rock head" friend was there.

He insisted on being there at 6 a.m. every day. He would get my report, then check in with my wife and daughter. Throughout the day and night, he would field all the visitors, calls, questions and food and drink deliveries to give my family a break.

"Whatever needs to be done, I will handle it," he told us.

Many times I told him that he could not afford to be there at my hospital 24/7. But he's a rock head and wouldn't listen.

Again, I learned to let others help you. It might help them get well, too. When you look past your pain to see someone else's, pride begins to melt into humility and you realize you are living for more than just yourself. Nothing empowers you more. And that's how it's been with me and my "rock head" buddy; best friends and brothers to this day.

Even after the deck that his crew built collapsed and nearly killed me one day. And now you know… "the rest of the story."

A GIFT AT THE DOOR

I had been home from the hospital for a month when the doorbell rang one afternoon.

With Sandi on the phone talking to our mortgage company, and me melted into the La-Z-Boy, we couldn't get to the door in time. Why only one ring? I rolled my walker over, stood up and moved to the door.

Sandi was on the phone because I hadn't worked for two months, and now the money was gone. I couldn't work, and I never would again; I just didn't know it yet. So we were scrambling to buy some time until we could figure it out. Welcome to the world of cancer.

We'd been so consumed with keeping me alive that other issues, including finances, paled in significance. Certainly the subject of money had come up in conversation with fellow church members and friends. They knew what a strain we were under.

But nothing prepared me for what I saw when I opened that door. I saw bags and bags and bags of groceries, household supplies, you name it. I was so overwhelmed I burst into tears. Crying was almost a daily event for me during that time. In fact, it still is. *And I hope I always remain broken enough so the tears can seep out.*

Sandi ran to the door, and we stood and cried together. We were so grateful. Whoever pulled this off had filled a huge need. I noticed the white corner of something protruding out from under the doormat. We pulled the envelope from its hiding place and returned to my chair where I immediately had to sit down again. Inside the envelope was hundreds of dollars in cash. *How blessed we were!*

Get this, fellow cancer warrior. Cancer can be a good thing – if you allow it to be. Through cancer, this stubborn, self-made man actually learned humility – and it made me a better person. *How important it was that I had recently encountered the young man with no legs.* If not, I bet my pride would have destroyed this wonderful moment in my life.

I was humbled again by a young married couple. They stopped by one day to hand me $100 from their own modest finances. They had discussed the idea with their pastor, and then given me the money they would usually have paid in tithe.

It's a powerful feeling to have someone hand you money, with no motive except to give in time of need. I didn't want to take it. My proud heart wanted to consider it simply a loan.

But remember that the giver is blessed by giving, not receiving. Don't let your pride destroy a very special moment in someone's life by not accepting their gift.

CREATE A LIFE YOU CAN LIVE IN

Alfred Montapert wrote, "The environment you fashion out of your thoughts, your beliefs, your ideals and your philosophy is the only climate you will ever live in."

Too long, I lived in the pathetic world of pride and selfishness. I know what it's like to live behind walls, unfulfilled and thirsty for love and truth, held by chains you've forged yourself. Your world revolves around you but it spins the wrong direction. The more you try to fix it, the faster and more out of control you become. You eventually form your perfect space with only you inside. Sad but true!

When my own storm clouds rolled in, they cracked open the climate of my little planet of self. The hurricane roared. My false foundations crumbled, and I fled to higher ground. And there I found the truth.

I tell you, make the choice. Look inside your heart. Are you spinning the right way? Leave your phony self-made hell. Experience real life and purpose beyond.

Warrior Words

There comes a point when a cancer caregiver needs information, mentorship and support. I now believe it is crucial to gain insights from another cancer patient other than the one you are care giving. Two hours spent with Jim was transformative for me. Getting an idea of how he felt and functioned through some of the toughest moments (although cancer treatment and side effects are very individual) allowed me to view Sherry's illness, abilities and fortitude differently. Jim shared examples from his own experience, using word pictures I could relate to, thus making it easier for me to communicate with Sherry regarding her illness. As a caregiver, I was flying blind, so to speak, and from time spent with Jim I had my eyes and heart opened to the cancer patient's view – and so much more. I would call it immeasurably beneficial! I only wish we would have had our visit sooner.

–Babette R. Banducci

CHAPTER 5
Sometimes It's Okay to Ask for Help

Junior high was a struggle for me. Things were out of focus and I always felt out of place. My family was struggling, my dad and I were butting heads, and my mindset was more on surviving life as a teenager than on succeeding.

I hated school and put in just enough effort to keep my grades up. That way, my dad couldn't find fault with that, too. Maybe he expected more from his only son and eldest child. My sister Janet, still in elementary school, seemingly could do no wrong.

On the other hand, I liked working. It seemed simple: If I did my job well, I got paid; if not, I was fired. I knew what was expected. And the money I earned gave me a sense of independence.

At a young age, I learned the value of work from my mom's dad, who we called "Paw." He brought me bruised fruit and vegetables, and I would sort them into little green baskets, line them up in my red wagon and go through the neighborhood selling them door-to-door. At 25 cents a basket, I could sell a dozen or so and I'd have some fishing money.

My dad worked as a driver for a courier car service, where I was hired to wash the entire fleet every weekend. By school's end I thought I had some pretty good money for a 9th grader.

CAN ANYTHING GOOD HAPPEN IN JUNIOR HIGH?

My worst subjects in school were English and spelling. *So now I write a book. Why not?*

Ninth grade was bad enough, but my teacher, "Old Man Oak," put it over the top. We did not like each other.

One day, angry about losing a race in track, about having to live at home and now, having to attend his stupid class, I let him know it. In return, he chose to move me to the far corner desk, the one for kids who needed an "attitude adjustment."

As I took my seat, a cute girl seated ahead of me in the last row of "good student" desks turned to say "Hi". I ignored her in my dark cloud of teenaged angst.

That Friday, Mr. Oak was all too pleased to announce a spelling test. I knew I'd had it.

And then, I hit the jackpot. I saw that girl in front of me was left-handed. By shifting my desk ever so slightly, being a "righty," I had a clear shot at her test. I knew these were "A-grade" answers I was copying, because the teacher was always praising her work. *Eureka! I thought. There is a God!*

She must have sensed my eyes across her paper. She turned her head as if to say, "Aren't you slick." When she maneuvered her paper even more to my favor, I knew that my grades – and my chances with the old man – had just taken a turn for the better.

I saw her again when I was walking home from track practice. She was standing on a front porch four doors down from my house.

"Hi Jim," she said.

"Where do you live?" I said, surprised.

"Right here. You live in that brown house, right?"

"Yes. How long have you lived here?"

"A long time, you?"

"Us too. Well, see you later." I turned toward home. As I glanced back, she waved at me.

I wasn't sure what to think. I was 14, and I was convinced I had too many cool things to do besides hang out with a girl.

But there she was, smiling at me again when I walked into the classroom to my corner confinement for another day in hell.

Sandi was her name. Her smile made her even cuter – and it still does, every wonderful day I wake up with my wife.

We were pretty hard to separate after that.

We'd share a Coke or walk home together. When I had practice instead, she would greet me as I passed her house. I found myself walking faster to get home. Before I quite knew what had happened, I was spending every minute of every day I could with her.

I even brought Sandi to my house to meet my parents, and I met hers. One evening after dinner with her family, Sandi and I paused on her porch. I grabbed her hand and thanked her for everything.

"I really want to see you more," she said.

I was nervous, but happy. It was wonderful to be around someone – besides my mother – who liked me, as screwed up as I was. I leaned forward and kissed Sandi right on the lips. Then I took off in a dead run for home, no stopping and no looking back.

I was soooo embarrassed, but, oh so hooked.

I fell in love with my best friend that night. From that first kiss in the 9th grade through today, I've wanted to be with her. Because of my rotten attitude, my atrocious spelling – and a schoolgirl's first shy smile in my direction – I found the love of my life. I guess I owe you a thank you after all, Old Man Oak.

TWO KIDS IN LOVE

Sandi and I had so much fun through high school. We knew we were more than just passing sweethearts. As we grew to be best friends, we shared a lot in common, both good and bad.

We needed the other's shoulder to cry on when our homes were in dysfunctional chaos. Both our dads, God bless them, were alcoholics. Our mothers put up with a lot of trouble to keep our families together, and for that we are both extremely grateful. We grew up fast. We had to, if we were going to break the generational chain and achieve what we wanted for each other. Our dads were good men who had made the wrong choice and set themselves and their families up for some rough times in life.

But in doing so, they also taught Sandi and me what not to do. *Thank you dads, we love and miss you both very much.* Both of our families struggled at times, living check-to-check and hoping to make ends meet.

Our sophomore year we wanted to go to a sock hop dance where costumes were required. We were so broke we couldn't buy any, so we handmade our own. We used the most worn-out Levis we could find, along with two of my dad's white T-shirts and some rope to serve as belts to hold our pants up. We were by far the most under-dressed, but I'm convinced that we had the most fun of any couple. We loved just being together.

That summer we both took on bigger jobs. I took a job at McDonald's, and every school break and all summer long I worked my butt off. Sandi had a job as well, and by teaming up, sharing and saving our earnings, we were soon driving a nice car to school. It even had an 8-track stereo!

I was really focused on vocational training, and excelled in wood shop, auto shop and my favorite culinary class. I loved to cook and still do. I wanted to have a good job the day after graduation.

I also loved track, and I gave it my all. I had won most of my one-mile races for our high school track team, but for some goofy reason, Coach Fletcher was more interested in my failing history grade.

"I can get that grade up to a D," I said, but coach was not impressed.

"Jim, you have a very good chance to place in the upcoming all-city meet, but I cannot let you run with that grade. I require at least a C or I will scratch you from the race. You have time, now get on it! Your team needs you in the top three if we are to win city."

I knew I was far from gifted in spelling – and definitely history, as well. The gift I did have was Sandi. The cool history teacher, Mr. Smith, knew we were going steady. Sandi had him first period and I was in his third period class.

I wanted a city meet medal more than anything, so I would get Sandi's history homework from her locker on my way to class. My work improved significantly. Still, I only received a C grade, and I asked Mr. Smith about it.

"Well Jim," he said with a smile. "That's all I felt you deserved. Since Sandi did all the work, I gave her the A."

Then came the night of the all-city track meet. I would compete in the mile-long race against the top eight runners in town. I was conscious of Sandi's eye on me as I took my place in the starting blocks. I was going to do my best to impress her. I wanted to hand her a medal.

The gun went off, and per my coach's plan, I hung back in second place until the last 50 yards. Those other guys were fast. By the time we crossed the line in a nail-biter of a finish, I'd come in third, passed up with just five yards to the tape.

I ran the fastest mile of my life that night, a 4:38, and our Hoover High School track and field team won the city trophy. Sharing my medal with Sandi, I realized I had won a lot more. She was so excited for my third place finish. I had always been told "If you're not number one, you're not anything." Instead, Sandi made me feel so proud. Wearing my letterman's jacket, she glowed as brightly as that bronze medal now hanging from her neck.

I stayed very busy with Sandi, school and the youth group at church. I was also working, running track and cross-country. I am proud to say I stayed with all of these things and in return, they made me better.

By our senior year, Sandi and I were acting like married kids. We just weren't living together. Everything else was focused on benefiting each other, both at the time and well past graduation.

DO ALL GOOD THINGS END?

The one and only time we broke up was the summer of our sophomore year. That's when a trusted friend of mine from school took off with Sandi in his souped-up piece of junk Chevy to chase a fire truck. Right! I knew this dog had eyes for Sandi; we'd had a run-in more than once over her. Sandi swore she had no feelings for George, but I was not so sure. *Why would she leave with him? Why has it been two hours? Okay, that's it, I'm sure our time is done. He can have her!*

When I saw his cherry-red car zoom past, I ran to her house and pounded on the door. Sandi's mom opened it.

"I need to talk to your daughter, now!" I said. Sandi came onto the porch.

"I'm sorry..."

I cut her off, "You hurt me and I trusted you. We're done!"

I left her crying on the top step. I was broken inside. I loved her and wanted to comfort her, but I was mad as hell.

My mom caught me storming back through my own front door.

"Jimmy, where's Sandi?" she said.

"She won't be coming down here anymore, mom. I just dumped her."

"You WHAT?" my mother said. "Are you crazy? You'll never find another girl as good as Sandi. Jimmy, honey, cool down and rethink what you have just done. You're jealous Jimmy, that's not good. You need her, our family needs her."

"But mom, she went with George!"

"Oh son, I love you."

That next week, Sandi's dad invited me to go on vacation with them to Lake Tahoe. I declined, but I did suggest one thing: "Bill, if Sandi wants to call me, she can."

It was the longest week of my life, waiting and hoping for the phone to ring. It drove me crazy. I wanted so bad to call her and apologize, but my stupid pride would not let me do the right thing.

Luckily, my sister Janet was plotting a way to get us back together. I drove Janet to the store on an errand, and she had hidden a surprise in the back seat – Sandi. We made up. My sister, bless her deceiving heart, had reunited what was meant to be forever. Sandi and I graduated together with the class of 1971 and were married July 10, 1972.

From a girl I didn't know existed just four houses away, to the only woman I have ever been with and the only woman I will ever be married to, Sandi and I have been inseparable ever since. Only once in the past 40 years were we almost separated again, during the cold winter of 2004 when I nearly died.

But long before that, we would find paradise together – our new home in Idaho.

NEW HOME, NEW BUSINESS

The stunning beauty of mountains reflected off a crystal-clear lake as a bald eagle soared in his peaceful domain. It was the spring of 1986, and I was staring once again in awe across Lake Coeur d'Alene.

This stop had become a ritual in my travels to visit my hunting buddy in Montana. Now that I was headed back to my home in hot, dry Fresno, California, I was more intrigued than ever by these cool waters and thick forests. I made a vow to myself: *Someday I will move my family here.*

The rest of my 18-hour drive, I worked over every angle in my mind. *It's a new goal. Can we do it? Where there's a will, there's a way.*

I kissed my wife hello, and called my kids to hear a hunting story over dinner. I also shared my plan: "I have a new goal. You know that place I talk about constantly? I want to move there. Let's spend some time in that area really looking around. What do you think, guys?"

TRUCK LOADED BUT FEELING EMPTY

It was our anniversary, July 10, 1992, on a beautiful Sunday evening in Post Falls, Idaho, ten miles west of my favorite lake. We spent the first night in our new home, after working all weekend unloading and unpacking, right on the heels of a two-day road trip from Fresno. *This moving is a real pain, but I believe it's best for the family.*

It hadn't been easy leaving. Sandi already missed her close-knit family and friends. She missed her mom and dad, who were dealing with his cancer. My dad had been court-ordered to live in a halfway house to rebuild his life. My sister had divorced and started life over with her three boys in Oregon.

And here I was, taking my family away from everyone in the wilds of Idaho.

My new job at a local HVACR company (heating, ventilation, air conditioning, refrigeration) started Monday morning in Spokane, Washington, 25 miles to the west. I loaded my truck with tools and got an early start, eager to get to work.

But the company owner sat me down for some bad news.

"I'm sorry. I had two full-time positions open when we talked last, but because work has really slowed, I only have one now and I filled it. When work picks up in a month, I really want you to work for us."

"What?" I shot back. "Are you kidding me? I just moved 1,200 miles from family, a very ill father-in-law and a good paying job. We unloaded everything we own in a new house in a town where we don't know a soul. You assured me I had this job!"

The owner said, "Listen, you are the best man for this job I have interviewed in some time. I'm very sorry Jim, I realize this puts you and your family in a bad way."

"I need this job," I said. "I'll even accept starting pay and work part-time."

"I can't do it," he said. "The work is coming but I can't hire you now. I'll call as soon as I can."

I went back and sat in my truck, sick to my stomach. *OH BOY! NOW WHAT? How do I tell my family I have no job? They're scared to death already. What have I done?*

Sandi and our children had made an incredible sacrifice for me to relocate here. I'd felt so confident about this move. I'd done all my homework and put years into this plan, but now I had no job. Driving around, getting lost for hours, almost in tears, I finally headed home to face the fire and brimstone.

I pulled over for a quick prayer. I had been so sure this was where God wanted us to be, but why? Now I was beside myself, thinking how I may have destroyed my marriage and family. *Still, if this is God's plan and his divine hand is over us, I have to trust him to make things happen and then do my part.*

I sat my family down at the kitchen table and explained what had happened. The kids began crying. Sandi jumped to her feet and yelled at me, "Let's load up a truck and go home!"

"Jim," she said, "You have a great job in Fresno. They'll hire you back in a minute. I miss my family. My dad is dying. Please, let's just go home. The kids haven't started school yet, so now's the time.

Maybe it's just not meant to be. I'm sorry, honey. I think it's the best thing to do right now."

I excused myself from the family meeting and went into the backyard. I kicked pine cones across the yard. I needed a minute to think and reevaluate our situation. My brain hurt and my stomach was sick. *Was I so selfish that I would put my family at risk of losing everything for something I wanted?*

On the other hand, I didn't think my family was safe in California anymore. My son Jeff had been jumped by other kids while walking home from elementary school because of his Chicago Bulls backpack. The junior high Kym attended had armed guards on campus. We'd taught the kids to run inside when a slow-moving car came down the street. I'd had enough of that nonsense. We'd moved north for a new start and a better way of life.

"Please give me a month to work things out," I told my family. "I will find a job, or I will make one."

So I pounded the phones, filled out countless applications, and took quite a few interviews. Problem was, $10 an hour after my 20 years of career experience wasn't going to work for me. And I didn't want to work out of town. I wanted to be a good dad. I wanted to be closer to home.

At one interview, the service manager, Brian, offered me a dirt-cheap wage. I turned it down. He took in my situation.

"If you don't mind me asking, Jim, what are you going to do now?"

After a pause, I said, "I'm starting my own company."

"Do you have a customer base to start with?" he said.

I thanked him for his time, and stood up to leave his office. Then I turned, "To answer your question, sir, the customers I'm going to have are YOURS!"

WE NEED A NAME

I brought my family around the table yet again. Following a short prayer, I explained my new plan and how determined I was to see it come to pass.

I needed to incorporate, and I needed a good name. With a base in North Idaho, I had considered "Mountain Air Conditioning and Heating," "Panhandle Heating and Air Conditioning" or maybe something with "Lake City."

My son Jeff, who was 10 at the time, said, "Jimbo, I think you are making this way too hard. When people are cold they are uncomfortable so they call you, and when they are hot they call you to make them comfortable, so I think the name should be 'Comfort Heating and Air, Inc.'"

When his little voice spoke that name it rang loud in my heart. I knew that was it. The company was born, so now what? I had $5,000 left in savings and a 1975 Ford pickup. *Do I risk the money on a new company? Invest it into parts and supplies? What if this fails and all is gone?*

Tough times bring the best or worst out of you. As my dad would say, "A turtle only makes progress when he sticks his neck out." I requested a separate phone number for the company even though I would be working out of my house. I didn't want my daughter trying to figure out why somebody's heater wasn't working! I also placed an ad in the local directory.

Within a week I had the truck ready, with big vinyl business signs for the doors, storage in the back for tools and supplies and a ladder rack on top of the shell. I started with the half section of a 22-foot aluminum ladder and a five-foot stepladder.

I had freshly printed business cards and freshly made work shirts with the new company name. I was ready to go – but where?

I drove my truck around town, looking for the service vans of that other company that hadn't wanted to pay me enough. I followed those vans to find out who their customers were.

Then I approached each one of those customers, introduced myself as the "new kid in town" and left my card. I told them, "If for any reason you're unhappy with their service, I would appreciate you giving my company a try."

The phone began ringing from my ad. With a few successful service and repair jobs now under my tool belt, I had some referrals beginning to come my way, which is the only work I really wanted.

I was waiting at a red light when I noticed the driver in the car next to me writing down my business number off the door sign. She called that night, asking for an estimate on installing air conditioning in her home. She had other bids but wanted one more.

I arrived at her home for our appointment six minutes early. She looked over my proposal and shook her head.

"Ah, Jim, you are much higher than the others," she said. "I'm sorry, but I feel led to hire another company."

Since this was my first estimate in North Idaho, I'd figured the job like we did in California. Oops! I asked to see her other bids, and sure enough, I was $2,500 higher.

I explained that I was new in town and just starting out, but that she could not find a better HVACR contractor than me.

I made her this deal: "If you'll allow me to install your new system, I will match the price you were going to pay with the other company. When my installation is complete and you are 110% satisfied with everything, you owe me that amount.

"I also want you to know that if you are willing to stick your neck out for me and my family, if for any reason you are not happy with my work or me, if you feel I cheated or that I've deceived you in any way, your system is FREE.

"Here's the catch: I will leave you with a box of my business cards. I need you to hand them out to anybody that has a pulse. I want you to refer my company because of the way I treated you and the quality of my work. Or, I want you to tell them how I screwed you over. Deal?"

She agreed!

That one installation set my new company up for what is to this day a referral-only business. Because she was willing to give me a chance, I was able to accomplish my part. Because of a red light, this gal made my business go.

Call it luck if you want – I believe that His divine plan was in motion that very day, at that very time, at that very intersection for that very job and beyond. I felt His hand on my shoulder when I would enter her home. Every Christmas, I gave her family a $150 gift card for dinner out, along with other goodies and gifts. She owned a lake house on – you guessed it – my favorite place, Lake Coeur d'Alene. Because of our "deal," she had a set of keys made so my family could enjoy it, too. *Amazing. Think about it.*

FEELING HOMESICK

Sandi had adjusted well to our new home, and seemed much more comfortable now that regular paychecks were coming in. The kids had settled into school. God bless them, it was a tough adjustment, especially for Kym, who was 14 and just starting high school. Checking to see how her homework was going, I would find her lying on her bed crying.

"Kym, are you okay?"

"I miss my friends, dad, but I'm okay." She hung in there for me, and I still owe her big time.

By now, I was working 50 to 60 hours a week. *Almost too much work!* I was not only doing all the calls and installs, but the business stuff until late at night.

And then John, the guy in Spokane, called to hire me, too. He was even willing to increase my hourly pay to what I was asking for. I had to turn him down, saying, "Sir, I realize this puts you in a bad way, but I own a company now. Too late."

I wasn't spending enough quality time with my family, but I had a great job, a growing business and I was home every night.

I took my homesick family back to California for the Christmas holidays, leaving a trusted fellow contractor in charge of my business. As the sole employee of Comfort Heating and Air, Inc., I needed help with my rapidly growing workload. I had a talk with Sandi's brother Gary, who was an excellent HVACR service tech. I asked him to consider moving to North Idaho and joining my company. For him, it was a big decision. For me, it was taking on even more responsibility. *How much angrier would my family be with me for this little stunt?* I would need to buy at least one more vehicle, maybe two, and fully equip them for the job. It would take a lot of money. *Now I had two families to support. Could this company do that?*

Gary did join me in the summer of 1993. Comfort Inc. was no

longer a new kid on the block. The company continued to grow, until we needed to move into a building space and hire another service tech.

In December of 2003, I had a moment of reflection as I pulled my new company van into my favorite view overlooking the lake. It was that same view that had prompted me to haul my family all this way and start over. Comfort Inc. was 11 years old and I had turned 50. I planned to groom Gary to take over the business, slowly slip toward more time on the lake and retire within the next 10 years.

I felt amazed and so blessed to call this beautiful location home. The lake still glistened under the unpolluted skies. My family had spent countless hours on this breathtaking lake, our boat gliding over the clean, cool water towing the tube behind, the kids holding on with white knuckles, screaming with joy. Sometimes I would fish for Chinook salmon or just cruise the shore looking at the beautiful homes. We'd take the boat back to the lake house to get some quality family time and work on our tans.

What was once only a thought was now reality. Records are set to be broken, and goals are set to achieve the impossible. Little did I know, but these accomplishments had put us exactly where I needed to be for my showdown with death, which was only a month away.

DON'T GIVE UP YOUR GOALS

When you take on cancer, it has to be a personal battle. Despite the help of your loved ones and your team of medical professionals, it all comes down to you – and how you decide to fight.

Each day requires a new commitment to succeed despite the odds. Every day's new mindset will determine what you accomplish that day. Some days, if you just stand up next to your bed you did more than yesterday. Good for you! Tomorrow stand up and take a step.

Cancer is utterly exhausting. As one dear lady told me, "There is no rest from chemo tired." Amen! Some days you will just want to quit. That's a choice you have every day, I want you to know that I struggled with giving up – but for only a moment. Then I decided that cancer would not be stronger than I was. Today I have life. Cancer may someday end it, but it will not be today.

My fellow cancer warrior, I want you to know that my heart feels your pain and depression. But don't give up. I want you to fight, to march ahead. I have always believed that if cancer kills me, it will be only because it hit me with a knockout punch before I could hit back.

Like a boxer, remember you need all the help you can get in your corner, but you must do the work. Consider every day as a new round in the ring. Fight to go the distance. When you get beat up, go to your corner and get a drink of water, a blood transfusion, a nausea pill or gummy bears. Have a good cry – whatever you need. Then stand up at the bell and fight. Your corner people want you to win. And so do I!

I BECOME THE CAREGIVER

One winter after we'd moved to Idaho, Sandi slipped on our neighbor's icy porch and broke her ankle. My business at the time was extremely busy, since winter in North Idaho is a good time to be a heating contractor.

When I got the call that she was on her way to the emergency room, I was angry, to be completely honest. How much time would this take? *I have a ton of calls today. Will I be working all night? I don't need this right now. And this is the best time to hunt geese. Will I have any time for myself?*

After surgery, when her doctor called us in to view her busted up ankle, I knew I was going to have to quit whining about what I wanted and step up to take care of my wife. The X-ray showed more screws and bolts in her ankle than I had in my service van. It was a severe break that would take time to heal. My wife, ready to come home to rest and heal, was going to need constant attention, something I am not good at.

Reaching our bedroom up the stairs was out of the question with the heavy cast on her foot. After much deliberation on how to pull this mess off, I built a bed for her in the living room, complete with a few layers of bricks from the yard, a piece of plywood, big pieces of foam and a spare mattress. I must say it wasn't pretty, but it worked great. It also seemed to be a good conversation piece when people would come over to visit.

Sandi spent six weeks in that bed. Because of the severity of the break, she was instructed not to walk, and to put absolutely no weight on that foot. Everything, and I mean everything, happened right there in our living room. *Till death do us part.* I remembered saying that 28 years earlier, but I didn't recall the part about washing out the portable potty, cleaning the vomit off her and the floor after the painkiller did not go down well, making her breakfast before mine, or running to the store for a "got-to-have ice cream" at 11 p.m. It took everything I had to take care of her, the children, my company and myself.

We had been "taken captive" by a broken ankle that could have, if allowed, destroyed our family, business and marriage. *Was it fair? Why my wife? Why in the best part of the winter and just before Christmas? Why not?*

My experience as a caregiver was enlightening. I had never really realized how all about me I really was. Having to wake up every day and worry, think about, and help someone who is totally dependent on you for a good day is tough.

When our children were small we thought nothing about our time or needs, because they were our life and we loved to be there for them. You knew that being babies, they were completely helpless without you.

I found that caring for another adult is much harder, because you think they are lazy, taking advantage, or just screwed up in their thinking from their own mistakes. It's hard to understand why the person isn't getting better faster. You feel like they should be able to buck up and get on with life again without you having to babysit them through each day. Both mentally and physically, it's very hard to cope.

Being a caregiver, in my opinion, is the hardest job a person can have. I am talking here about your spouse or family member who is also "taken captive" against their will, to care for, say, a stage 4 terminally ill cancer patient. If you're a good caregiver, it utterly consumes you, your time, thoughts and wants. Nothing is about you anymore.

Thank God for all you professional caregivers who have the compassion and heart to take care of others. By choice, you give yourself and your gifts to those who need attention, along with a friendly smile or a hug from someone they can trust. Thank you one and all, especially those who have been there by my side. I admire you, but I can tell you I would never have the strength to do your job.

During my wife's recovery from her broken ankle, the hardest emotion for me to overcome as her caregiver was anger. I guess it's against our basic instincts to put someone else's needs before our own.

I had important company issues to deal with every day. Instead, I had oatmeal to make in the morning. Then it was time to get the wash water ready for her sponge bath. By the time I changed the bedding and her clothes, it was lunchtime. And since I wasn't able to get to the store the day before, we had no variety for lunch.

While I was cleaning up lunch, my wife informs me of her doctor appointment at 4 p.m., and tells me she has no clean clothes to wear because I didn't get the laundry done. Well, that was because I was on the phone with the employees and getting us new jobs to be able to buy the clothes that I did not wash. After hearing the doctor remind us, "no walking for another four weeks," I had to stop to buy new pain meds and lunch stuff. This was followed by a "relaxing" evening of dinner, dishes, medications, ordering parts, house cleaning, serving dessert, business calls, getting her ready for the night, paperwork and payroll, finding the stupid remote control, feeding the dog, scheduling the crane for the lift in the morning, and last but not least, having to sit up with her all night because she felt safer with me by her side. *Whew!*

Well, we got through it together. I stayed by my responsibilities until my wife was ready to walk again. The kids did a great job of helping mom and each other. My wife was truly grateful for the care and concern, and gave us credit for her healing, even though I know she "did the work." My company and customers survived, and I was a better man for looking past me to see someone else.

I didn't know it yet, but the cared-for would soon become my caregiver.

THE ROLES BECOME REVERSED

Lung cancer was not an event I had on my bucket list. I never thought how cool would it be to experience chemotherapy just once before I died. And then it took me captive. In the very same living room where I'd been forced to take care of my wife during her own ordeal, I sat miserably in my La-Z-Boy and tried to hang onto life.

Sandi was working at the elementary school three blocks from our house. After getting me settled for the day, if that's possible during the days of chemotherapy, she would be off for her work day. She would call me every hour to check in.

We needed her at work because my job was over. My son was at college two hours away and my nurse daughter had a full-time job and a husband-to-be. Most of my days were spent sleeping, and – you guessed it – reading the Book of Daniel.

My dear wife never missed a chemotherapy treatment. She went with me to every single one for a year and a half. Her employer was very understanding and willing to make do without her. I tried to accomplish what I could around the house, but what should have taken an hour took four hours, so I was very little help. Sandi would come home for lunch and check on me, refill my ice and water, restock my gummy bears (my go-to food for nausea), give me my medicine and refresh my new office (recliner chair) where my work now was simply to live. She would blow me a kiss, go off to finish one job, and then come back home to her tougher job, me.

Three years earlier, I had become a caregiver – against my will, I might add! Now, watching my wife work herself to exhaustion for my needs, I realized I would never have had the patience with her or my family had I not served my caregiver apprenticeship.

With God in control of all things, I believe the progression of our lives is in order to teach us and build us up. During the lesson, we think it sucks and it usually does, but He knows what your future holds. Without this test now, your faith may not be ready for what is coming next.

When I was the caregiver for my wife I learned I could not be selfish and that I needed help. Now my wife was doing the same for me. We were now both prepared to face our futures together, unselfish and without pride. *With that mindset, what can stop us?*

My wife, God bless her heart, was such a marvelous caregiver. She was so much better than I was to her, I'm sure. My condition became such that she resigned from her job to stay at home with me.

On those days when I just wanted to quit, I was so thankful she was there. Hugging each other and crying were daily events. We were both so overwhelmed by the thought of being separated. Sandi named these days "Crybaby Days." We would both cry and cry like babies, sometimes not even knowing why. But this sadness in our hearts brought us closer.

I want you to know that "Crybaby Days" are a must if you are going to be a survivor. Just promise me you won't stay there!

We would cry together, talk things out, discuss death staring us in the face, hug and hold each other. Now that's a caregiver. Your caregiver may not know the medical terms or conditions or even what to do for them. But when you're a patient, just like when you are a child, love is spelled TIME.

It was a long, tough haul but we made it. We are both richer for the experience. If you are the cancer patient, who is your caregiver? They may be family or they may be professionals. Either way, I hope you treat them right. I hope you thank God every day for them being unselfish enough to put their lives on hold to extend your own.

WHY AM I ALIVE?

It's been nine years now, and counting, since I had just two hours to live. *I often think, why am I alive?* That's a very complex question and one I know I don't have all the answers for. But I can tell you what I know.

Without a doubt, I am alive today because my higher power, Jesus Christ, wanted it that way. I must give credit to Him to whom credit is due.

Although this world does not show it well, God is in control. The Book of Daniel emphasizes the sovereignty of God. I believe he controls even the day I was born and the day I die, just like He knows the numbers of hairs on your head. That said, I have two cancer survivor friends who can't even spell Jesus who are alive today after impossible odds.

The realization that I should be dead keeps me focused and humbled like never before. Still, I'm no angel. I am in constant prayer to help me stay in tune with His plan for my life. Here's the truth: If I do not discipline myself to stay focused on the miracle that God provided for my family and me, I would very quickly drift from plumb and be redirecting my own plan for my life.

We all know (I hope) that our plans will end in destruction if left up to us. Even after all the grand lessons taught through the trials of this life here, and after witnessing God at work in our lives, we, by our crooked nature will default back to what we know and that is Self Induced Nonsense, or S.I.N. *You need help from on high!*

THE BEST CAREGIVER OF ALL

Through my struggle with cancer, my wife's broken ankle and countless hard times with other families who have allowed me to be a part of their struggle with whatever, I have come to realize again and again what a wonderful caregiver we have in the Lord. He is everything a caregiver must be. He is loving, patient, unselfish, forgiving and most important, He is always there when we call out in distress. Not judging or condemning us, but by love, wanting to speak a kind word into our hearts to comfort us and to give encouragement when the end seems near.

You may ask "Why would The God of All Things want to give peace and rest to my soul when I really haven't been close to His plan for me?" Or you may not believe there is a God. Either way, your cancer may bring you to a place where now you need a miracle and you don't want to die. I suggest you call upon God as you know Him and ask to be saved.

Your will may have to change if you want to live. Even if you don't make it, dying with no regrets will bring peace to you and others. I believe He works through the direst of circumstances to strengthen us so we will go out to strengthen and encourage others. I believe that's why I am alive today, to give glory to God and live for others. *What else is real?*

It is such a blessing to give credit to others, to be humbled enough that your pride can be overruled by the fact that you needed help, asked for and received. To be able to stand tall and admit that without help, *I am not here.*

In our culture it's against the grain to show weakness. "Oh come on," we want to say. "Man up. You can beat this thing. Don't be weak! You are tough enough, you can make it happen." When I hear someone say that to a loved one, I know they have never had cancer.

Because we have been brainwashed about asking for help, we go through life trying our best, which isn't much, to show the world how tough and independent we are. My fellow cancer warrior, I want you to know that cancer does not show you're weak. It's a pride breaker. If you allow it to, it can clear your vision. You must open your heart and focus on others to see the real life that God wants to extend to you.

Swallow your pride! Ask others to help you. It shows you're a candidate for a miracle. *Why would God help me? Why not?*

Warrior Words

Dear praying friends and family,

Yesterday was eleven months exactly since I heard my diagnosis of cancer. I saw my oncologist for the last time. He has resigned and is moving to Sacramento, California, to be with his wife who is at U.C. Davis working on a doctorate in nursing. He has been commuting for the past two years. I will miss him, but I wish him well. I have not met my new doctor yet, but I trust the Cancer Center to make a wise decision in hiring a new physician.

As usual, my blood counts were perfect. In all the time I've been receiving chemo there was only one occasion that there was a problem. He has continually told me how well I am doing, and my nurse tells me constantly that I am the "Poster Child" for how chemo is supposed to work. I have only been sick a handful of times. I've had very few days of nausea, and no vomiting at all. I have not had issues with tiredness. In fact, I seem to have increased energy. I went kayaking for the very first time earlier this week. I had such a good time I plan to go again tomorrow.

Yesterday I heard the words I didn't expect to hear. At this time my oncologist considers me to be in remission. I am still far from being done with my treatments, but it is all worth it. I will be continuing to receive Herceptin for a minimum of two years. At that time I will reassess my progress and go from there.

Phil. 4:19

–Love, Tracy

Dear Friends,

Today is the one year anniversary of hearing I had cancer. I thank you for your faithful prayers. If it were not for you I would not have gotten through this past year as well as I did. Before anyone knew I had cancer, God was already at work calming my heart and uplifting me. I didn't have to work at trusting God to "get me through it." It never entered my mind to be afraid. Maybe I didn't realize how serious my diagnosis was, or maybe God so overwhelmed me with His grace and comfort that there was no room for fear. Each day I would wake up and say, "I trust You God with my day and whatever it may bring."

I celebrated my 54th birthday this past July; a milestone I did not expect to reach. It was a special occasion for me as I was even more aware this year that none of us is ever guaranteed another birthday.

God is leading each of us day by day and step by step. He is the one who gives us the strength to get through each situation. God does not want us to run from our problems, but to run to Him with them. They are not mistakes; something God did not know about. They are a chance to experience a blessing from God. We do not know what the future holds. The future is a secret thing and secret things belong to the Lord. All we have to do is trust God because He does know the future and that is all that matters.

God has promised to meet all our needs according to His riches in glory. It has been a good lesson for me to learn that what I consider to be important may not necessarily be what God sees as important. I have to remember that God has said to us that His ways are not our ways and His thoughts are not our thoughts. I will understand fully one day when I meet Him face to face. Now all I have to do is trust in Him.

As most of you know last month my oncologist told me he considers me to be in remission. I praise God for what He has done in my life and thank Him in advance for what is to come because God has only my best interest in mind. It is not possible for me to need something that God cannot do.

I thank you for your continued prayers as I continue along in my journey.

–With a grateful heart, Tracy

CHAPTER 6
The Wisdom of Fellow Warriors

What a day! I had a salesman waiting in my office, a service van that wouldn't start, an office heater that wouldn't heat, a lost cell phone and a full schedule of service calls. And it wasn't even 8 a.m. yet.

I rushed to the phone that was ringing off the hook at my desk.

"Jim, it's Val," said one of our dearest family friends. "Don and I really need to talk with you and Sandi. Can you make it over soon?"

"Val, is everything okay?" I said.

"Well, he went to see the doctor yesterday. If it's at all possible, can we talk, please?"

"Can it wait till noon, Val?"

"That's fine, see you guys then. Thank you."

I didn't like the tone of her voice, and my stomach was in knots. The things I'd been pulling my hair out about just a moment ago now seemed trivial.

Don and Val had become great friends of ours. Don and I were hunting buddies, and Val and Sandi were "Bunco Babes" and worked together at the local elementary school. Our children played on the same high school teams.

We soon learned Don's news: He had stage 4 colon cancer, which had metastasized to his lungs. We felt helpless and sick to our stomachs.

This was March of 2003. The trouble had started the previous fall, when Don returned from a successful moose hunt in Canada feeling ill. He thought at the time that perhaps he'd just had some bad water. I knew him as a tough partner in the backcountry. Now, to see him so weak and frail was quite depressing.

By the summer of 2003, he was well into his fight and holding steady. He knew a lot about cancer already because of his previous job as head of the pharmacy department at Kootenai Health, where he was now a patient.

He had tremendous confidence in his oncologist, Dr. Tezcan. They had worked together for many years on the cutting edge of cancer research. He knew Dr. Tezcan was doing everything possible to help him win this battle. In turn, I knew Don would do his part to win. I committed myself to do mine to help him.

A year earlier, Don had booked a goose-hunting trip in Canada. Despite how sick he felt he was still determined to go.

Some days he could barely walk; others, he would just stay on his couch, read, watch TV and try really hard to find that all-elusive "sweet spot" to get some sleep.

Even so, he overcame the objections from Val and I, and insisted that Val drive him to his hunting partners home to begin the hunt. He was as stubborn as an old mule; that's what I loved about him the most. I remember Val pouring him into the front seat of their car and hooking up the seatbelt to keep him upright. He gave me a very frail wave and off they went.

I'm not sure if it was when Don vomited blood or when he passed out that Val finally decided to bring our strong-headed, determined friend home and get him back to his couch. I admired Don's attitude. I remember thinking: *If I ever got that sick, would I have the same determination to live life?*

The next day Don called my office with a special request.

We spent the rest of that afternoon together watching goose hunting videos in his living room. Instead of lying in Power Hunter blinds, surrounded by 100 goose decoys in a snowy field, we admired our feathered friends from the comfort of our couch.

I'll tell you what – we really enjoyed that time together. In fact, Don and I agreed that his living room that day became the best goose field we'd ever seen.

Welcome to the "new normal." Cancer brings change, but life goes on if you want it to. Find a way!

That day brought joy, but also sadness, knowing that our real field trips might be over forever.

At Don's next monthly check-up in November of 2003, his markers were higher. His medical team could not capture or contain the disease, and he was running out of options. Our couch discussions now focused more on God, life and family than ever.

Don became even more determined to accomplish the goals he had set before him. His daughter was getting married in June of 2004, and attending her wedding became his ultimate goal. At this point, I knew the odds were very bad, but I also knew my friend was a tough cookie. He would do whatever it took. As I watched him fight and not back down, Don continued to be a real inspiration to me. Even though he was in constant pain, he was a tremendously positive influence to everyone around him.

Don and I would soon become partners in the fight of our lives. I just didn't know it yet.

He was excited when I told him about our upcoming hunt – the last one of the season. We were taking the duck boat down to the southern bays of Lake Coeur d'Alene.

He warned of the heavy snow predicted, and gave us a bit of hunting advice and his good luck wishes.

"Take lots of pictures of the ducks," he said.

"You got it, my man," I replied "Are you going to be okay? Val has my number, so you better call if you need me, you hardhead. I'll visit you on Monday to let you know how we did."

It turned out I would not keep my promise to visit him for another two months. By that Monday, I would be in the ICU myself, instead.

HUNTING BUDDIES TURNED WARRIORS

Now it was Don's turn to be in shock over the news of *my* diagnosis.

He wanted to visit, but he was so sick he couldn't leave his couch. Just sitting up, his wife told me, was his way of "having Jim's back."

The first time he called me was a day I will never forget. We cried on the phone for five minutes before either of us could say a thing. We were physically and mentally spent, filled with fear for what might be ahead. Finally, I found words to speak.

"Don, let's go hunting."

He chuckled, and our new journey was off and running. That day, we went from hunting partners to cancer partners. Life is strange, but in my opinion I couldn't have found a better warrior to go to battle with than my old hardheaded friend.

Both of us believed that God was in control. We accepted what he had allowed, and "made up our minds" (Daniel 1:8) to fight together. Our faith in God was our sword, and our friendship was our shield. We would stand tall, and march, crawl or roll to victory.

After my two-week stay at our beautiful "medical hotel" ICU, I couldn't wait to see my cancer soldier, but I could barely move. I wanted to share with him what had happened to me that night I'd read the Book of Daniel. As a man of faith himself, I knew it would encourage him, give us strength and help us depend on God and not ourselves.

It took two months before I felt strong enough to get out of my chair to go visit. Struggling up the staircase myself now, finding my couch next to his, I began to talk to Don in a whole new and powerful way. Cancer has a way of humbling, and if you could have been there to see and hear two grown men cry and call out for help, I know you would have been moved like I was. *Overwhelming!*

And then my friend gave me his game plan for my survival. In his "spare time," he had made me his list of "Dos and Don'ts With Cancer." I was so fortunate to have Don as my mentor in those very early days of the disease. He started me out on the right foot.

WALKING MIRACLES

I have some heartfelt advice for you if you are in a fight for your life:

Get help early! It's so very, very, very, very important! Swallow your useless pride and find a friend. Nobody can understand you like a fellow cancer patient can. Having the right person to talk to, cry with and share the agony of cancer is huge. Find your mentor!

Don was there for me. He was more concerned for my well-being than his own. He looked past his pain to mentor me. And what gave me strength was being there for him.

As my mentor, Don could answer every question I came up with. I remember calling him early one morning, concerned that I had woken three times in the night lying in a pool of water. Sandi had changed the sheets twice.

"You're having night sweats," Don told me. "Yep, you'll have them a lot. Nothing to worry about."

Time and again, he talked me through my problems using the everyday, firsthand wisdom that I needed. Cancer knows cancer, and having a mentor – and being a mentor – is an absolute must.

Don was a very private man. I was very honored to be invited to share our cancer struggles together. We would share thoughts and feelings that would only be spoken between us. There is a special understanding between people who have faced cancer face to face.

He and I made a point of talking every day. Whether it was good or bad, the key was talking about it. We starting setting goals that we would challenge each other to make:

Who could get the best cancer marker number that week?

Who could go to the bathroom on their own more times?

Who was going to gain more weight this month?

From there, we started getting serious about life and living. We set some goals that seemed impossible with the odds we'd been given.

At the top of our lists was the fact that our daughters were both getting married that summer. We talked about this goal a lot. Both of us felt good about our future sons-in-law, and wanted to be there to give our daughters' hands at the ceremony. Problem was, those weddings were months away. That's a long time when you're not even sure about tomorrow. We shed some more tears together.

What if? What if we couldn't pull off this impossible task? What if our wives had to walk our daughters down the aisle? How painful would that empty spot in the family photo be? What about that first dance?

The talk of the weddings would have been, "If only your dad could see you now," and "Your dad would have been so proud." That was heavy stuff to contemplate.

We knew staying alive for those weddings was a long shot. At times during these discussions, we could barely crawl off the couch long enough to throw up.

"It would be easier for us to go elk hunting than make these weddings," Don said once. We laughed. But when your life is focused on being there for someone else, you gain a special strength.

Don did indeed make it to his daughter's ceremony, and he walked her down the aisle. It took tremendous strength and determination. By now, he had to wear an infusion pump all the time, and flying across the country was no easy feat. But he did it.

I wish I could say the same, but it was not to be. With my severe deep vein thrombosis, low blood counts and defenseless immune system, I was unable to fly – and deeply disappointed. While my mentor achieved his "impossible goal," I was back in the infusion room again.

I was the first one to demand details of the wedding. Sharing the photos together, my buddy and I were back in our favorite "goose-hunting field" again.

And then, it was Don's turn to root for *my* daughter Kym's wedding. Better yet, he was able to attend the ceremony. One miracle in a lifetime is more than most people ever see. And here at Kym's wedding, there were two miracles walking around. Everyone knew it and the mood reflected it. Together, we enjoyed a very special evening that I know will be cherished forever.

Once again, God proved that a small seed of faith could move mountains. Both my cancer mentor and I had been blessed far beyond what we deserved.

And then it was October of 2004, and Don and I began the very painful discussion of quality versus quantity. My mentor had fought the good fight, but the disease had taken its ugly toll, and there was not much left to do. My hero was fading before my eyes. The reality was nearly impossible to bear. I honestly wasn't sure that I could go on without him.

Through the tears of a broken heart, I encouraged Don to enjoy what time he had left.

"Do what is best," I said. "I will support you no matter what."

The treatments were done. He gained back a bit of strength and pep, but not enough to stay out of the Hospice ward. His family gathered around him. I visited every day, and I made sure his family knew what a wonderful help Don had been to me.

One morning I went to his room very early for some quiet time with Don. He told me I was his "angel" and that I gave him strength. This remarkable man was encouraging me even while he was dying. He tried to raise a cup of water to his lips, and failed. I helped lift the cup. With our eyes locked, I was lost for words to thank him enough.

I laid my head on his shoulder, and I hugged what was left of my friend.

"You are a miracle, Jim," he whispered to me. "I want you to remember that. I want you to be accountable."

I kissed his forehead, and then my mentor was gone.

He passed to the better life on November 2, 2004. It made me despise cancer all over again. And I made a promise: Until the end, I will always be accountable. My mentor told me so.

WHAT IF THE CHEMO ISN'T WORKING?

Maybe you are receiving chemotherapy as you read this. Maybe you're wondering, *"What if?" What if after all this sickness, pain, down time and depression, there's nothing but more bad news?*

Believe me, I understand.

As a cancer patient, I found it hard to stay focused on good thoughts. Honestly, most of the news I received at the beginning was all bad – really bad. It took me a while to become comfortable with the fact that there is no quick fix for cancer. You can't just see the doctor and get this or take that. It's more than just "drink it, rub it or eat it and then check back in a month." I realized that I could be dead in that month.

Never in my life had I experienced anything like chemotherapy. It doesn't just attack the cancerous cells – it attacks your whole being. It holds you captive and tries to control your every thought and emotion. It destroys good and bad – it has no favorites. It will, if allowed, render you helpless. But chemo cannot affect who you really are, deep down. It cannot steal your faith.

When cancer aims its target at you, you need your own missile lock. You need a resolve to live for something beyond yourself. On those days when you just want to die, you need to look into the faces of your family. In their eyes, you'll see the pain they feel about losing you. Their pain can be the anti-venom for yours. Their pain will clear your vision and give you the mindset you need to defeat the enemy.

Living every day with cancer can continually haunt you. *What's this? What's that feeling or pain?* On the other hand, waking every morning is such a gift, even on chemo days! The only other choice is a lot less painful… but it's a "dead" end.

In the early days of my cancer, I had tremendous doubts. I would become so nervous that I would actually make myself even sicker. I worried constantly. *If the chemo didn't work, slow down, hold stable or hopefully shrink the tumor, then what?* It was very hard not to think the worst.

That fateful morning in the ICU, the pages of my Bible looked as dim as my future. And then I came across that wonderful story of three courageous young men. Daniel and his fellow captives would give their lives before they would bend to what had brought them into captivity. They would not waver from what they believed.

These words rang through my desperate mind: "If we are thrown into the furnace, the God we serve is able to save us from it. And he will rescue us from your hand, O king." *How amazing! Listen to what I read!* "But even if he does not, we want you to know, O king, that we will not serve your gods or worship the image of gold you have setup."

I remember how these words flooded my soul with warmth, hope and strength. In that dark hospital room, it was like that story was shedding enough light to help me see the end of the tunnel.

I was overcome with emotion. I realized in that moment that *it did not matter* whether or not the chemo was working. It was not that I had lost hope of survival – not at all. Instead, I knew my faith would see me though this dark and painful time. Even if the chemo did not work to slow or eliminate the cancer, I would hold true to my beliefs and push on. I would be a witness to my family, my doctor and others.

KEEP DOING WHAT YOU LOVE

I changed my attitude to believe I could beat this foe called cancer. I decided I was going to live life. I was going to do everything my doctor told me to do, whether I liked it or not. I was going to be involved with the functions going on with my family and church.

I want to encourage you – *do those things you did before cancer.* Don't let this disease take them away. Sure, you might need to adjust your mind to the new slower speed your body is moving now. But take your throw-up bucket with you, and go on your outings anyway.

There were times I went to graduation parties and other events so weak I couldn't lift a glass of water – but I was there. People who knew my condition were blown away that I could find the strength, that I could walk the talk. I was so determined to go to a men's breakfast once that I went in a wheelchair. I was hurting the whole time, *but I was there!*

I went fishing when I was so sick I could have never reeled in a fish. My family, bless their hearts, would help me to my chair on the dock. At that point, it had nothing to do with fishing and everything to do with doing.

Don't let other people do the work for you. You must do it yourself. I remember having 20 loving, caring people wanting to help me get a drink of water. Instead, I got out of my recliner. I crawled, rolled or walked to get my water. Your caregivers can help beyond belief – but in the end, you must do the ultimate work.

There is no neutral setting with cancer – you're either in forward or reverse. There is no tie – you either win or you lose. You must fight for each day. You must have a clear purpose. You must have power.

"Are you kidding me?" you might say. "I can't even get out of bed to go pee. What power?"

Well, do you believe in miracles? This book you are reading is a miracle. A "dead man" wrote it – and lived it! And if I lived long enough to write this book, you can live long enough to read it, and then write your own.

Early on, I made up my mind that I would not be tortured on my deathbed by regrets. I gave it my all, even when it appeared the treatments had failed, and even when I had more bad news than good.

So what? I would say to myself, and to the cancer. *I am still alive. I will push on through whatever you throw at me. Hey cancer, you've got the wrong bull to ride. I am going to buck you off.*

LIVE OR DIE? YOU DECIDE

I remember well the first time my doctor told me that the cancer was back and I would have to start chemotherapy again. After nine months of treatments, I really needed a break. I had a constant sick feeling in my stomach, and eating was no fun when everything tasted like a piece of sheet metal. The only two things I could even tolerate were orange sherbet and gummy bears.

After 50 years of life, nothing had been more terrifying than having my CT scan or blood marker show that bad things were coming. Each round of my fight with cancer seemed to get tougher and tougher. I remember how weak I felt, how worried and scared of what lie ahead.

I also remember the comfort of my pastor sitting beside my bed. I'm sure he felt as helpless as I did.

"Flourish in captivity instead of feeling forsaken," he told me. We discussed the fact that even though the chemotherapy was not working, I still had faith in myself, my future, my God and my family.

Cancer will test your faith, in whomever or whatever that may be. And by experience I can tell you this: Your faith had better be in someone who is stronger than the cancer.

I can't say I flourished through all that comes with cancer and chemotherapy, but I can say that I did stay loyal to my commitment. *I wasn't bucking very hard or high, but I will always keep bucking.*

And that was only the first of three very discouraging relapses before I finally reached the relief of complete remission. Every time the report was bad, my family and I would regroup and rethink our battle plan, discuss options with my doctor and settle into a new course of action.

HOW YOU CAN MANAGE

Cancer is worse than you can imagine. Only cancer patients know what cancer is like and what it takes to survive. But if you've just started your battle with cancer and chemotherapy, I want to share how I managed.

The first thing you must do: Decide if you want to live or die. That's easy to answer before you begin treatment. Believe me, you will change your mind after a few bouts with chemotherapy or radiation. Certainly, it would be easier to die than to live with the fatigue, night sweats and vomiting – and may God help you when your blood counts go down and you need "the shot." After that shot, my bones ached and sleepless days and nights were standard affairs.

Believe me, my friend, it's a tough war, but you can win it.

Today, we have some of the most advanced cancer medicines known to man. Trust your doctor, his plan for you and his advice. Trust your faith, yourself and your loved ones. Most important, do your part!

Never let the cancer curse go eight seconds on your back. Buck it off with everything you've got, which on some days will be nothing. Nevertheless; "make up your mind." Come hell or high water, stand by your commitment. Do you have one?

Cancer will expose you from the inside out. It will magnify your smallest weakness. Cancer will test you by the pain and fear it brings to see if your heart is in tune. You – and everyone within shouting distance – will know once and for all what you're really made of.

Your previous life with all its accomplishments or failures means nothing now. Cancer could care less how you look, who you think you are or what you own. Cancer does not see you like the world does, judging by outward appearances. Instead, it looks straight to your heart, where real strength resides – along with the ability to defeat this rotten disease.

Outward beauty, money, career, big houses, cars and anything and everything else you might have worked your rear off to get mean absolutely nothing. They cannot and will not help you now. This war will be won or lost on how strong you are on the inside.

And maybe for the first time in your life, like me, you will realize how precious life is and how blessed you have been to gain all you have, especially when it's all in the correct order; that is, from the inside out.

Your victory over cancer can show you a brand-new perspective – an understanding that real life is the only good life.

Now you can experience real love, real friends, real beauty, real wealth and real family. You can share what you have been through with others.

Here is my prayer for you: Make up your mind to experience the real life that cancer will give you in return for your hard-fought victory. You *will* emerge as a stronger and better person, and I can assure you this – you have now been remade from the inside out. *Enjoy!*

SEEING IS BELIEVING

I remember a night in the hospital, tossing and turning with pain that was out of this world. Two years into my battle, I'd just had the cancerous tumor removed from my lung.

My nurse came in to check on me, and I invited her to pull up a chair and stay a while. It sure was better than talking to myself at two in the morning! She noticed that I kept feeling my stomach.

"Is something wrong there?" the nurse said. "Mind if I take a look?" She gave my stomach a closer examination.

"Oh my," she said. "That's a very large bump. What is it?"

"It's a tumor," I replied. "A cancer tumor."

"But I'm confused," said the nurse. "I thought they just removed a tumor."

"Well, they did," I said. "This one just showed up."

"How do you keep up the fight?" she asked with tears in her eyes.

I smiled with determination. "I have made up my mind to win this battle and I will win."

"What are they going to do about the new tumor?"

"Well," I said, "I'll go back on chemo when I get strong enough to start up again."

She looked down for a moment, then said, "What if the chemotherapy doesn't stop it from growing?"

"Listen," I told her, "I will always remember this night, your concern for me, your tears and your time spent with me when I really needed help."

Then I sat up and gave her a hug. Through my tearful eyes I looked into her own tear-filled, compassionate windows to her soul.

"I want you to know," I continued, "that even if the chemo does not work, I have been allowed to have this moment in time with you. We have blessed each other. Talking about the ups and downs of life with you has brought peace and calm to my pain.

"The Lord can deliver me from this new tumor by any means he chooses. But even if he does not, I will stay to my commitment, calling things that are not as though they were. That's faith."

I saw the same nurse again in the hall, months later.

I smiled again, and lifted my shirt to show her my stomach. There was no bump. There was no tumor. Seeing is believing, and so is touching. She put her hand on what had been that large lump, a place that was now tabletop-flat. She smiled back at me.

"You said it," she said. "You said even if it didn't work you would keep your faith."

And how is your faith, my friend?

DON'T GIVE IT THE BENEFIT

Two years after my successful lung surgery, now in full remission, I wanted to sit down and talk to the surgeon, Dr. Burnett, who'd performed what I'd been told was a very high-risk procedure. We had spoken in passing, in the halls or riding the elevator in the hospital together, but now I scheduled a one-on-one.

I was anxious to hear his opinion on my case. I wanted to know why he had undertaken such a feat. And I wanted to thank him for his work.

"You had to do your work, too," he said. "My part took three hours and your part took two months. I was amazed at how well you recovered and gained your strength back."

He continued, "And don't thank me alone, Jim. You should really be thanking my professor in medical school who taught me, 'Never give the tumor the benefit of the doubt.'

"Because of your attitude and desire to live for you and your family," my doctor said, "I remembered my professor's words. Up until your case, I'm not sure I even considered that quote. But there was more to you than just the tumor. The safe way was leave it alone, but I decided not to give the tumor that benefit of the doubt."

I will forever be grateful to him for his courage to step out of the boat and perform a very risky task, against all odds. He believed in his heart and in himself.

It's a good lesson for everyone, but especially for you, my cancer warrior. Never give your cancer the benefit of the doubt. Don't ever surrender. *Thank you, doctor, for helping me. Now I pray I can help others.*

WAITING FOR THE HELICOPTER

My daughter, the nurse, told me about a patient at her hospital. She'd shared my story with him, and he'd asked if we could meet. I came to his hospital room.

Through the pain of my own cancer, I could see the weakness in his body, but also the joy in his spirit. He was in dire need of a heart transplant. He spent each day waiting and wondering... *What if there was never a heart to replace his worn-out original?*

One day, he stopped me in mid-sentence.

"Jim, do you hear that?"

"Hear what?" I said.

"Listen, listen! It's coming in."

Thinking my weak-hearted friend might have been staring at the ceiling a little too long, I told him I didn't hear a thing.

"It's closing in, Jim," he said.

I looked out his window, not sure what I was looking for. I turned to tell him he was imagining something. And then, there it was, a helicopter that circled the hospital and landed on the roof three floors above us.

"How in the world can you hear that thing when it's a mile away?" I said.

"Jim," he told me, "I've been in this room for three months now. I know if I'm going to get a heart it will arrive by helicopter. I hear every one of them that lands, day or night, because I know one of them will be delivering my heart."

I was blown away.

"How many land in a day?" I said.

"One, three, sometimes none," he said.

"How do you do that?" I said. "How do you keep your hopes up? You've been here around 90 days. If just two helicopters land per day, that's 180 times that thing has landed three floors above you. And not one has brought your heart yet.

"How do you stand it? Do you ever lose faith, or just say, 'Well, I guess I will never survive this. Time will run out before I will receive a transplant?'"

"Jim," said the man who needed a heart, "let me tell you something, I know that God is in control of all things. You can agree with me or not. I know there's a plan for my life. I've had a wonderful life and I wouldn't change a thing. But I do know that there will be a helicopter landing on this roof with my heart as its precious cargo. And I will be made whole.

"So I listen for each one as it comes within the range of my ears. I pray it's my heart, but regardless, I pray for whoever has just arrived."

Wow! I wanted to stay there all day and listen to this guy.

"I have been very blessed," he said. "I've been blessed because I kept the faith, blessed by not doubting God or myself, blessed because my family visits me every day and we talk and share our lives more here than ever at home.

"My helicopter will come, but even if it does not, I have been blessed with life and will be blessed in death."

Amazing! I glanced at the time, which had passed so quickly that day.

"I must go now," I told my new friend. "Thank you for encouraging me and sharing your faith. And by the way, I do agree. May I come again to visit?"

We shared a hug, along with a prayer for him and his family, and off I drove to another appointment. I was on fire inside, knowing that nothing is impossible. And when you're a cancer patient, that's always a good thing to remember.

The very next day, his wife called with joy in her voice.

"I wanted to tell you that the helicopter has landed."

My friend, can you hear yours?

THE SECRET TO SURVIVAL

If you only get one thing from this book, I suggest that you burn these five words into your heart: "Even if it's not working."

I believe those words hold the secret to survival, no matter what holds you captive.

Even if it's not working, I want you to keep watching for that helicopter.

Even if it's not working, I need you to be strong.

Even if it's not working, you must be true to your beliefs. You must be transformed from the inside out. You must do the things that matter most.

This attitude will get you through the shadow of death, which as a cancer warrior is a shadow that hovers overhead 24/7. Remember, this shadow itself cannot hurt you, although it sure can cause doubts and "what-ifs." *Oh boy, will it ever!*

114

You may go through the burning fiery furnace itself, along with Daniel and his loyal friends. Only when they were fully exposed to the heat did their real resolve shine through. (Daniel 3:18)

They knew they would be safe from the flames. But "even if they were not," they would stay strong and faithful to their cause.

And so can you and I.

Warrior Words

Why is it when a man feels he's got everything under control it all falls apart? My name is Tyrell Monette, and two years ago the Lord used a single picture in a hospital to answer that very question for me.

A little background history on myself: I graduated from Post Falls High School in 2000, moved to Murrieta, California, and graduated from Calvary Chapel Bible College in 2005 with a degree in Theology. I moved back home to Idaho the summer of 2005, and by Christmas I had met the woman who would later be my wife and mother to our daughter.

In 2008, with a daughter on the way and no extra money to buy baby furniture I decided to build it myself. After two months I had made a crib, dresser/changing table, rocking chair and nightstand. With some wonderful compliments on what I had made and a newfound love for building cabinets and furniture, I decided to find an apprenticeship with a cabinet maker.

Okay… it's 2010 and I was three weeks away from my wedding date. I had a beautiful little girl named Kloe who was very much in love with her Dad. I was at work by the table saw when I dropped my pencil. Reaching down to pick it up I felt a POP! Not able to catch my breath, I called my father to come take me to the ER, where we discovered my right lung had collapsed.

They poked a hole in my chest, inserted a tube and sent me home. Now remember, this was three weeks before my wedding! A week later, after a failed attempt to re-inflate my lung, I was admitted into Kootenai Health Center. Another week went by and they still couldn't get my lung to inflate. The doctor sat down with my fiancé and I and explained that even if they opened my chest up and try to find the hole in my lung, they still might not be able to make that lung work.

I remember trying to be as strong as I could while my fiancé and daughter were in the room with me, and I remember the devastating feeling as soon as the door shut behind them. Two weeks ago I'd been set to get married in a castle to a beautiful women with the prettiest flower girl that ever was… and now I didn't even know if I'd be able to leave the hospital on my own two feet or without having a vacuum pump attached to me wherever I went.

I remember falling to my knees beside the hospital bed in tears, crying out to the Lord and telling him that I could not do this on my own. It's amazing the power of the Holy Spirit to bring scriptures to the front of your mind, little jewels that I had forgotten long ago. I don't even know how long I was broken on the floor but I remember the nurse coming in with a wheelchair to take me down to X-ray. This was the X-ray that was going to determine if I would be in surgery the next morning or going to walk down the aisle in two days.

Right before the nurse took me into the room she got a call and had to leave me in the hallway. My knuckles were white from gripping the wheelchair handles so tight. So many thoughts were going through my head. I thought, "the wedding is already paid for," and I thought about my daughter crying because I was not going home with them.

That's when I looked up and saw a picture of Jim Morrison, posted by the Kootenai Health Foundation on the wall. I remembered hearing about him in Bible college from his son Jeff, about his diagnosis of cancer and how long they gave him to live and that by the mercy of Jesus Christ his cancer was in remission. I'll never be able to explain the peace that came over me as I stared up at Jim's picture. I remember thinking that if the Lord could bring Jim from a death sentence with six months to live to cancer-free, then healing my lung was nothing. No matter what, the Lord would use this experience for His glory.

The next day I walked out of the hospital and a day later, I walked down the aisle. The spontaneous pneumothorax (collapsed lung) that I had suffered from has not returned nor have they figured out why or how it happened.

I know why… The Lord had to bring me to a place where I could rest on Him, receive from Him, respond to Him and rejoice in Him.

–Tyrell Monette

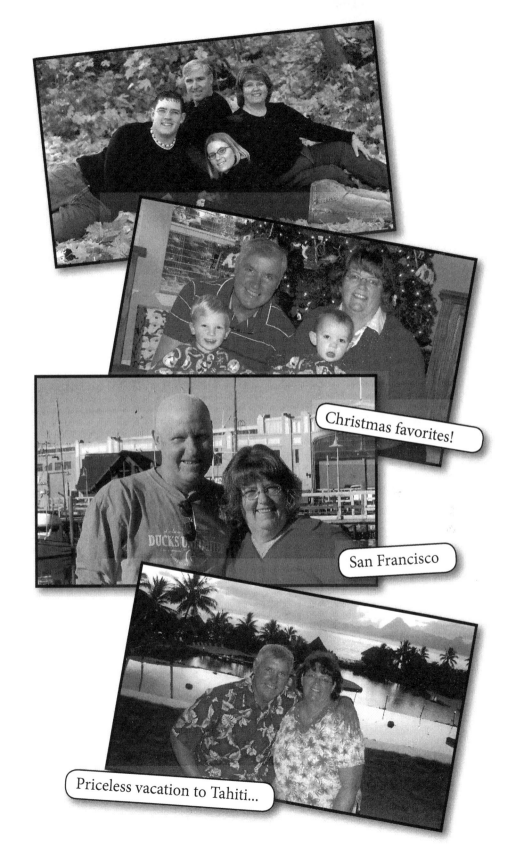

Christmas favorites!

San Francisco

Priceless vacation to Tahiti...

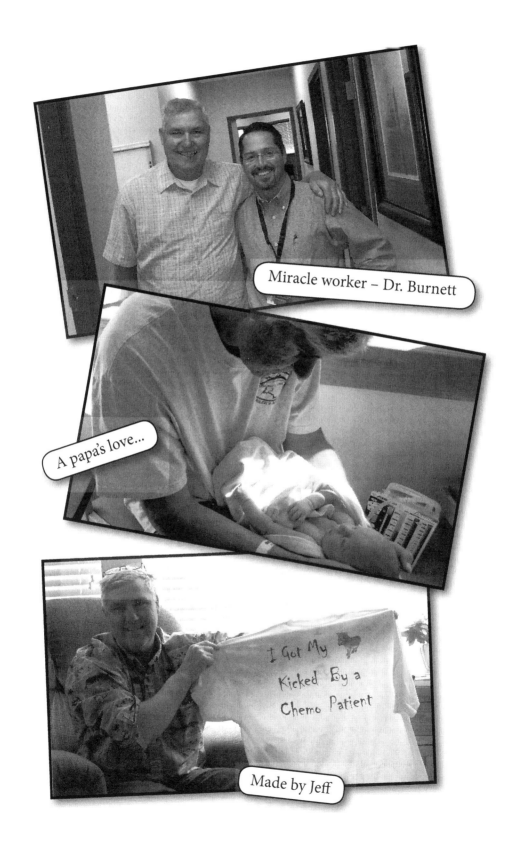

Miracle worker – Dr. Burnett

A papa's love...

Made by Jeff

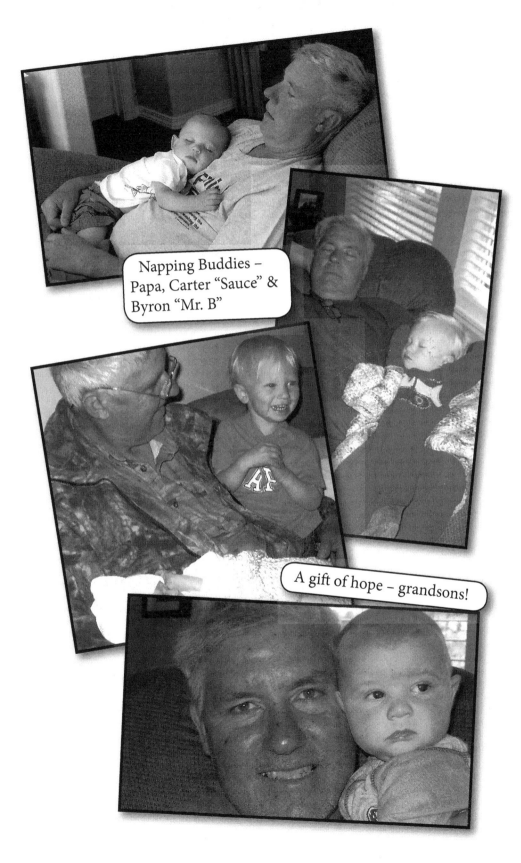

Napping Buddies –
Papa, Carter "Sauce" &
Byron "Mr. B"

A gift of hope – grandsons!

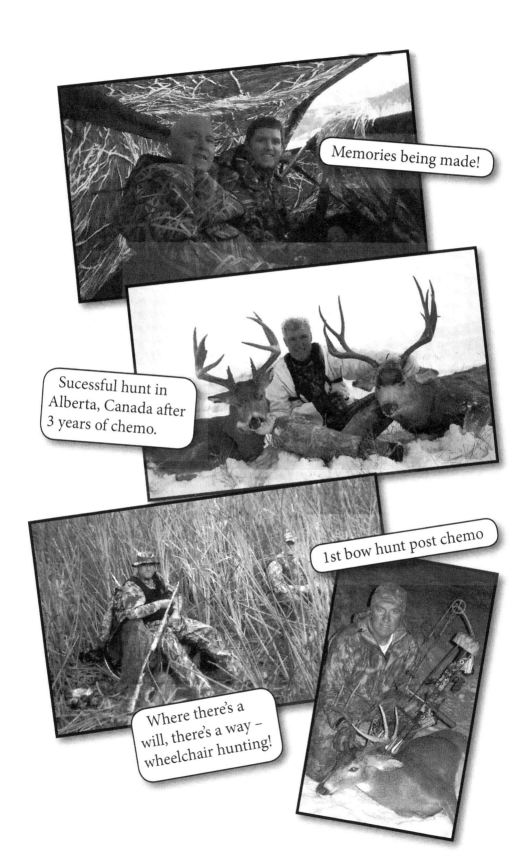

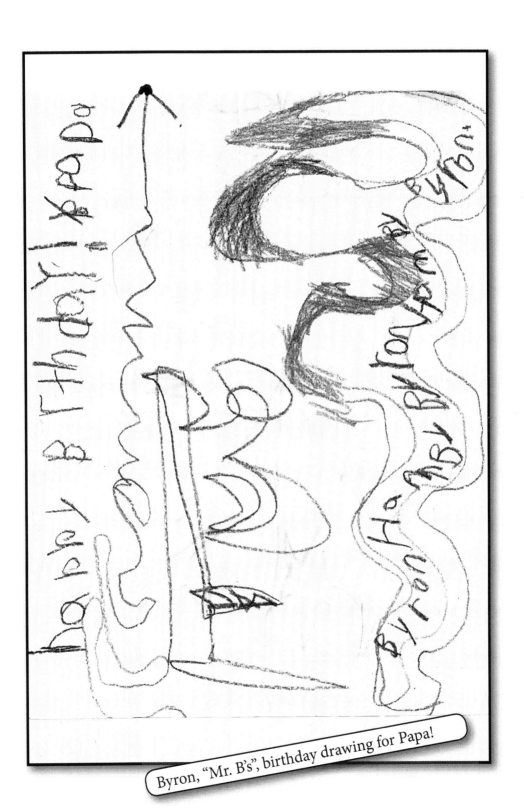

Byron, "Mr. B's", birthday drawing for Papa!

CHAPTER 7
Enjoying Life's 'New Normals'

As I write this, it's been eight years since my diagnosis of stage 4 lung cancer. I have been in remission now for five solid years. Yes, I am a blessed and happy man – blessed by the things around me, and happy by what I feel within me. I'm still alive against all odds.

Along the way, however, I've had to adjust to what I call "new normals." The collateral damage of three hard years of chemotherapy and medical procedures, along with five more years of living with cancer, has changed my day-to-day life significantly.

These past eight years have included three relapses and four surgeries. I have had numerous blood transfusions, received booster shots for my blood count and have lost all my hair three times. I have had a Gunther Tulip™ Vena Cava filter placed inside my body to block the severe blood clots forming in my legs.

My gall bladder was removed. So was half of one of my lungs. In a pericardial window surgery, doctors opened the sac around my heart and drained the fluid so my heart could keep beating. I had two chemotherapy ports implanted and later removed, along with a surgery to remove a six-inch piece of the port tube that had broken off inside my chest.

I still endure an IV contrast as part of my regular CT scan. This is a dye injected to help the scan, and when it reaches my chest and heart I get an intense warm feeling and a sick metallic taste. I'm still paying my dues. Every day I feel the effects of cancer in at least a dozen ways.

I'm not looking for sympathy here. I'm just being honest with you: when you beat your cancer, the war will not be over. New battles arise every day. You will have to adjust to "new normals."

But the best news is, I'm alive. And so are you – so let's get on with living. *Amen!*

WHAT ARE "NEW NORMALS?"

Nearly all the cancer warriors I know agree that fatigue is the worst side effect of chemotherapy. "My get up and go has got up and went" is a daily complaint. To be honest, it was at least a year and half after my final chemo treatment before I started to regain any strength. So hang in there.

The fatigue never seems to let go. A simple task can take hours. It's so frustrating for your mind to know how and what to do, only to find your body in another zip code. I've found that any strenuous job or task must be tackled first thing in the morning when I'm at my best. Usually by mid-afternoon, I'm out of battery and in very urgent need of a recharge.

My legs also feel very heavy and tired by this time of day. Even with the full-length compression stockings I wear, I must elevate them often.

At some point in the day, I lie on my back with both legs elevated well above the heart and connect my sequential compression device (SCD), which pushes fluid up my legs to the lymphatic drainage system. This brings much relief and really rejuvenates my legs.

I'd never in my life given myself a shot anywhere. Now, every night before bed, I inject my blood thinner medication. The side effect from this is, well, sex. If you know the mechanics of a man's erection, you can figure out why a blood thinner might cause a malfunction.

The cancer-fighting pill, T-100 Tarceva, that I thank God for every day (my "pill and a prayer" routine), also has some "new normals" to go with it. Sometimes it makes me itch from head to toe throughout the day. Other times, my stomach growls constantly, so loudly that my wife can hear it from across our living room even with the grandkids playing. In quieter settings it's a real problem.

Another side effect of this pill is facial pimples. Actually, it's pimples all over my body. Those can be embarrassing, even on a good-looking stud like me. *Ha!* This pill also makes my face get very red and flushed – even more so in the summer heat.

But those are not the worst effects of this life-saving pill. It also makes for a very loose and runny bowel movement. No kidding, some days I sit on the throne six times or maybe more. When I travel I pack diaper rash cream – what a relief!

This little white pill has caused me so much misery, but along with faith, and doing my part, it has also extended my life. I thank God and man for its invention. I'm even grateful for the side effects. Why?

Because it shows it is working.

WELCOME TO THE WORLD OF CANCER

My fellow cancer warrior, I'd rather you hear about these "new normals" from me than from a website or a medical expert.

Like me, you might need prescription glasses after chemotherapy. I'd never worn them before – and it's another thing I've had to get used to with cancer.

Chemotherapy caused my fingernails and toenails to become very brittle and fragile. They needed close attention and constant trimming. My mouth stayed dry all the time, and the ringing in my ears was so loud sometimes I couldn't fall asleep. It's a miracle to me that I've been able to recount my experience in this book, since I also suffer from the foggy memory I call "Chemo Brain."

I live with these things every day. You may have to deal with some of them, or you may not. Don't panic!

I just want you to know that even after years of remission I am fighting the good fight. I will fight cancer, or its side effects, for the rest of my time on this earth. I want you to be prepared to fight at the beginning, during and after your bout with cancer.

CAN I ENJOY LIFE NOW?

When I was in the hospital for my lung surgery, it was July of 2005. There is a fishing derby on my home town lake which my brother-in-law Gary and I have participated in for over ten years. We have even won money and great prizes with our salmon we caught. It was always held the last week in July. I'm told this surgery was a bear and it could take time to recoup. Could I be ready by derby time?

As the days drew near to fishing time I had my doubts, but I was determined to talk my doctor into releasing me in time. Day after day I begged, but it fell on deaf ears. Finally he'd had enough.

"Jim," said the doctor, "If you want to chance going out in a boat on that lake you are crazy. I will not release you because of your weakened condition, not to mention two chest cavity tubes that would allow the lake's cold water to flood your lungs if you fell overboard. Absolutely not!"

Looking out the second-floor hospital window toward the lake on opening day of the fishing derby was the first realization that life was going to be a whole lot different from here on. Just one thing made missing that day on the water special. As I was looking and wishing to be out there, my newborn grandson, Byron, was cuddled in my arms and buried against my painful swollen chest. He had fallen asleep on my shoulder, and in his peace, I found mine.

WHO DO YOU THINK YOU ARE?

One summer, I met this guy for a cup of coffee at the suggestion of a mutual friend. Two days earlier he'd been told he had cancer. We traded small talk about the weather and baseball, and then he complained about how cold the coffee was. He asked our waitress for a steaming hot refill, took a drink and threw a fit, yelling, "Now this damn coffee is so hot I can't drink it!"

At this point, I was ready to leave. In my experienced opinion, if you can't tolerate the temperature of your coffee, whether too hot or too cold, you are in serious trouble when it comes time to deal with cancer. The rest of our conversation went rapidly downhill. Everything I brought up he already knew about, yet he did not even know the stage of his cancer nor had he once stepped foot in an infusion room. He criticized me for bringing up all this "doom and gloom."

"I have had a tough life and cancer will be just another bump in the road that I will cross and then get on with things," he said.

Our waitress came back for coffee refills, and as she swung the pot his way, he refused, saying harshly, "No more lukewarm coffee for me." I felt like telling him that I could already see the blister forming on his upper lip. For my part, I was grateful just to be out and about on a nice day. I was going to enjoy my cup of coffee, no matter what this guy had to say. Absolutely nothing that came out of his mouth was helping him or me. And then he stopped mid-sentence and looked me right in the eyes.

"Who the hell do you think you are to sit there and give me advice about victory, when you're a full-blown alcoholic?"

Aha! I knew right away what he was thinking. And yes, I do have a flushed face, but as you now know, that's a side effect of my cancer medications.

"Are you done?" I asked him.

"It takes a lot of balls to talk like you do, you wino," he told me angrily.

"Look," I said. "You're right! It does take a lot of 'balls' to talk to as many cancer people as I do, and I'll tell you why: Because some of them are going to be dead in a year's time.

"You bet it's hard. They have the same disease I have. Why do I want to be around cancer patients? Why do I want to see the Hospice care, or deal with all the grief-stricken family members who have come to say goodbye? Why do I want to see what my future might be?

"I already experience helplessness every day in my own fight. Why share in theirs? It breaks my heart when the grandson is crying on the bed next to my precious cancer friend.

"Hey, I'll tell you why I talk to cancer warriors. I do it because it encourages us both to fight and do the best we can. And by the way, you really don't know it all – or know anything for that matter. The reason this 'alcoholic' you're dealing with has a very red, flushed face is because of the pill I take to survive cancer and not become another statistic. When I'm exposed to sunlight it makes me glow like Rudolph the Red-Nosed Reindeer.

"So you have a problem with coffee? I want you to know that if we are to meet here again in a year's time, you'd better change your attitude from a prize horse to a stubborn mule."

I saw him again two months later, but our meeting was very different. He was flat out on his bed, and he never even knew I was there. His family members were very kind to me for stopping and discussing his progress. They told me he was really struggling with the chemo and that it was worse than he'd expected.

"He told me he just wants to die," his wife told me.

"Please call me if I can be of help in any way," I said. Over the next few months, I called many times for updates, but he wanted no visits from me. Eventually his wife did call and she invited me to his funeral. It was a nice service – and I should know. I go to a lot of friends' funerals these days. It's one of my "new normals."

THE DAY I TACKLED A THIEF

One day after my chemotherapy treatment, Sandi wanted to go to Shopko, which was right across the street from my cancer center. It was a beautiful sunny day. The chemotherapy sometimes made me feel very cold inside, so I asked Sandi to park where the sun's rays could penetrate the windshield onto my body. It seemed like a great place for a nap.

Just as I was getting comfy, I noticed a young man running out of the store with a security guard dragging behind him. The guard had hold of his backpack in such a way that the man could not shed it or the guard. I was pretty sure the guard had caught this kid shoplifting and in trying to apprehend him had found himself in a real jam.

Cancer or no cancer, "new normal" or not, I had to help. I got out of the car, walked up behind the kid and hit him with everything my cancer-ridden body could produce. I knocked him flat, I jumped on top of him and held down the only arm he had free. As the guard worked free and got ready to make his move, I got clobbered right in the face by the kid's recently unbound arm. Now I was mad.

"I'm a cancer patient who just got my treatment," I yelled. "I'm in no mood to put up with a lowlife like you." I stuck my elbow with all my weight on it deep into his Adam's apple.

The young man's face was turning blue. I let the guard pull me off, and he handcuffed the suspect. A crowd had gathered around.

I walked into Shopko with the guard, the backpack and the handcuffed kid, and we went right past Sandi in the checkout line. Her eyes gave me that look I know so well: what did you do now? I guess it was obvious I hadn't just stuck with my nap like a good boy.

Well, I got a new pair of glasses out of the deal. My son came up with this idea for a T-shirt I could hand out to future "victims," reading, "I Just Got My Ass Kicked By a Chemo Patient."

CRAZY BUDDIES ARE A MUST

After my first remission, my son Jeff and my brother-in-law Gary came up with the brainstorm to take me duck hunting. At that time I could walk maybe 50 yards on flat ground before I collapsed, exhausted. We drove three hours through beautiful scenery, and then took a boat ride up the river. Just accomplishing those feats made for a successful day as far as I was concerned. They loaded me into my wheelchair and began pushing me across this mud bog full of cattails, slow but determined to get me into their hunting blind. They were really working hard to make this day special.

At some point, they lost control of the chair and dumped me, along with my gun, lunch bag and decoys into the muck and mire. I was a bit upset, although I'll admit it was hard to tell because I was laughing so hard. *Okay guys, I'm ready to return home to my La-Z-Boy chair and get my legs up now.*

They said they'd done it in love. Isn't that nice? They kept pushing, and together, we had a day that only a cancer patient and their family could appreciate. Those guys got me back in that chair and on with the hunt – although I noticed something interesting. They were way more interested in taking pictures than they were in shooting birds. I'd never noticed their keen photography urges before. And then I figured out what they were up to.

Of course. This could have been our last duck hunt together. I have cancer. It kills. They wanted this day to be forever in mind and on paper.

Before cancer, I used to carry bags of decoys, my gun and a stool for a half a mile through mud twice that bad with chest-high waders on. Those days are gone. Do I quit and stay home in my chair and have a pity-on-me party? Not on your life! I have been given the gift of extended time. It was hell to earn it, but I will accept my "new normal." I will make a point to enjoy life more now than ever.

ONE STEP AT A TIME

I greatly enjoyed deer and elk hunting before cancer took it all away. *Or did it?* One day I noticed my hunting bow in the basement. I hadn't even been able to pull the string back for three years. Would I be strong enough now?

You'll never know how many times I'd thought of selling that bow for the cash we so desperately needed at times. But here it was. I gripped the bow, attached my release and began to pull the string back to anchor. And, yes! I reached full draw.

My eyes began to water just thinking about the possibility of hunting again. Then reality quickly slapped me. With no strength in my legs and only one and a half lungs, how would I climb in the mountains? *Never say never.* I began searching for a ladder stand that I could set up against a tree and sit while watching a trail or crossing for game animals. I wasn't sure I could even climb a ladder, but it sure seemed easier than hiking around in my condition.

With months to go before opening season, I had time and persistence on my side. Every day I'd practice shooting the bow, and try walking a little further to build my legs. With a little help from my hunting partners, the stand was ready to go.

Our family is blessed with a beautiful home on five acres in the woods. This is where I would renew my hunting passion. There was one benefit – my wife Sandi, who previously had to worry about me hunting in the middle of nowhere with no cell service, could actually see my tree stand from her kitchen window!

I was thirsty for bow hunting again. *Enough of this chemo and sickness.* Hunting and fishing had always been such a great part of our lives that I absolutely refused to allow cancer to steal them. What a wonderful experience to be outdoors again. The pursuit is the same, while the technique is a "new normal." But I can tell you that I enjoy every moment of it in a brand-new way now.

That first time back in the woods, I honestly could have cared less if a buck ever set foot within bow range of my stand. It was incredible just to be able to climb those 12 steps, sit in my tree stand and enjoy the peace and quiet of the forest. *Are you kidding me? I've just come from a place where if I could bend over to get my shoes on it was a damn good day.*

For me, hunting has never been about the success of the kill. Now, it was all about killing the cancer demons that through the dark days kept whispering in my ear: *It's over. You're finished. The cancer will deplete you to nothing, and you'll do nothing ever again.*

I did get another dose of the "new normals" when I went to Idaho Fish and Game to get my hunting tags and signed my new disability license. With cancer, everything becomes a new milestone during your journey – some are bad but more can be very good.

It was impossible to think of what used to be, when just three years earlier, I'd buy a sportsman pack that included every tag under the sun for hunting and fishing. With my energy at the time, I'd chase 'em all! Now I was grateful just to purchase a single tag, which I knew good and well had little chance of being filled. *Sure it's a "new normal," but it also comes with a new life, thank God.*

As I sat in my tree stand that November, I noticed a movement to my right. Very quietly, a nice buck was walking the trail. From 40 yards away, he moved cautiously to 30 yards and then closer still. When he was 20 yards away, I released my first arrow after three years of chemotherapy.

The joy of another accomplished goal filled my heart with joy and my eyes with tears. I could see the buck lying on the ground, felled by my arrow. I cried out loud, another "new normal," overwhelmed by this moment in time that I doubted would ever come to past.

If you're under the heavy weight of chemotherapy as you read this, I love you and feel your fear. I know what it's like. But please listen to me: Pay your dues! They will enable you to someday climb to wherever you want to go. Then you can look back on your chemo days and marvel at how wonderful your "new normals" really are.

MAKING POSITIVE "NEW NORMALS"

What could be positive about cancer? The word alone immediately drains you of hope and puts out the fire in your soul. Of all the diseases known to man, I am most terrified of this one. Positive news can be hard to find.

Even when you have a good check-up, is it really positive? As I write this, there is no sign of my disease. Should I ignore it like it was never there? I don't think so. I am always on the lookout for the enemy, for I know it is very persistent.

Cancer seems like a predator. It never sleeps, and it is cunning and relentless. Many times I have actually felt that it was stalking me.

Will it strike again? Why? How? Where? Have we killed our enemy or is it just reloading? Will we find it in the same position or has it changed course? Will there be any warning first or just a full-blown attack?

Even though I deal with this train of thought every day, I refuse to give in to fear. I talk and write positive because I am. I have faith because I know who holds my future in His hands (Daniel 5:23). Still, I deal with clear-eyed reality.

You must take the negative of cancer and make it a positive "new normal" in your life. Find your newfound strength and a new appreciation for life. With the right mindset and attitude, you can enjoy "new normals" for which many people would love to trade their mundane, status quo life. I remember how that game was played, because I played it, too. I remember thinking that my life would be grand if only I could have this or that. We think that by working, lying, cheating or throwing whomever under the bus we can achieve the prize at any cost.

The bliss and excitement carry you for a while, and then you feel the emptiness in your heart resurfacing. You can't believe that you have been deceived again. You're chasing the dream everybody says will make you happy, but it is only smoke. The wind blows and it's all gone. You gain everything, but have nothing real.

Don't go that route, my friend. Let cancer help you make that change. If you're going to chase something, then chase real dreams with positive gains. These real dreams will not only benefit you, but help others to achieve their dreams, too.

A positive life is good for you and the world.

NEW LIFE!

My brush with death gives new meaning to my life, and everything that pertains to life. I'm living it and loving it with all the energy I can muster. I believe that this new life with my "new normals," this second chance I've been given, is the real thing we're all searching for. It's ironic that we never find it in the pleasures we pursue, when all the while the pain of illness holds the secret.

I enjoy life now in a whole new way. There's a new value to things; new dreams to achieve, a new urgency to make good choices and to mend broken relationships immediately.

Here's something else I'm thankful for: I now have a new filter to strain the crap on TV and the Internet. I now sift everything until one or two very small, meaningful things fall through, but oh, how important those small things are now.

I have no patience for the nightly news and entertainment drivel, for the media's version of "what everybody's talking about," or for "must-see TV." I don't care. It's not my reality. These days, I find myself much less interested in what the Right and the Left are saying, and more in who's right and who's wrong.

My loved ones and I are in our own "reality show" with a real drama called cancer. When my grandsons say "Hi Papa," there are no more powerful words spoken in the world. A piece of notebook paper with my name written in crayon by a four-year-old is more valuable than gold.

I'm even grateful for toilet paper. Very soft toilet paper. Due to the side effects of my medication which create frequent and runny stool, I have stashes of my favorite toilet paper brand everywhere you can think of.

I encourage you to keep working to make your own "new normals" positive ones. I know that for me it was very difficult at first to connect all the dots on this new adventure, but before long the image was clear and direction certain. It's a great feeling.

For me, it's better to live with some inconveniences than not to be alive at all. That's a positive thought! When I run out of energy now, I tell myself it can wait until tomorrow. My patience has become infinitely better.

My "before cancer" days are gone forever, and in some ways I'm glad. To be truthful, it's taken many years to accept this new direction and the things that are missing from my previous life, both good and bad. But I have embraced my "new normals" in a positive, constructive way, I am happy, blessed and eager to experience the miracles of the life I have left.

You are welcome to come along. *Can you keep up?*

Warrior Words

We were all devastated when we got the diagnosis of Jim's cancer. Then imagine my further shock when I was diagnosed with stage 2 breast cancer. The family didn't need this! We needed to be concentrating our prayers and efforts on Jim. I was sure I couldn't be as strong as Jim was. He is such a pillar of strength. Even with all that was going on, I wasn't scared of losing my breast to cancer, because I'm more than the sum of my parts. I'm a woman because God made me that way, not just because of body parts!

Throughout this trial, I've learned a lot of things from cancer:

#1 – God is in control, not me! Look at Job, what he went through and how he kept praising God. Even when his wife said to curse God and die, he didn't.

#2 – God's mercies ARE new every morning (Lamentations 3:22-23). Through the Lord's mercies, we are not consumed, because His compassions (mercies) fail not, they are new every morning. Great is Your faithfulness.

#3 – Don't assume plans. God has other ideas and His plans are better! Even with cancer!

#4 – There can be a lot of joy in trials. James 1:2-4 says, "Consider it all joy my brethren when you encounter various trials, knowing that the testing of your faith produces endurance. And let endurance have its perfect result, that you may be perfect and complete, lacking in nothing."

#5 – Enjoy family and life every day. It's beautiful!

#6 – You really don't have to sweat the small things!

But remember most of all – God IS in control, so you don't have to be! Relax in Him! Also, I would like you to know that I'm cancer-free, and have been a survivor for going on seven years now. I prefer to be called a conqueror! Romans 8:37 says, "Yet in all these things we are more than conquerors in Christ Jesus."

–Julie
Jim's sister-in-law

CHAPTER 8

Before and After Cancer

Yes, I'll admit I love heavy metal, even though it's the music my parents said would corrupt me. If this is your favorite music, too, I'm guessing you were as shocked and saddened as I was on May 16, 2010, to hear that the metal legend himself, Ronnie James Dio, had passed away.

I've been a loyal fan since I first heard his soaring vocals on the album *Holy Diver* in 1983. In my opinion, he is the all-time greatest singer in heavy metal history. His physical stature may have been small, but his act was bigger and better every time I saw him perform. His battle with stomach cancer closed the curtains on his act with no encore, his brilliant career cut short by a killer with which we are all too familiar.

Oh, how I despise cancer!

The idea behind this chapter came one day when I was working in my shop, listening to a song by AC/DC. This book isn't meant to offer a "quick fix to cancer." If you know one, please share it with me! Rather, I wanted to share the good, the bad and the ugly of my own battle with this disease. Eight years have passed since I became sick. I have five years of remission and my doctor is requiring only two check-ups a year now. That's amazing. Since I am blessed to still be here, performing on the stage of life, my goal is to encourage you to perform to the very best of your ability. I will continue to share my story until my last show.

I began thinking about what cancer has changed in all areas

of my life. I would argue that change is unavoidable, but also vitally important. No matter where you are in your courageous fight with cancer or any other captivity, if you want to win you must find change within. Yes, there may be change in your outward appearance, but it's the changes on the inside, the important side of you, that will bring victory. If you want it, it will come from within. *Trust me, I know!*

Here's my list:

BC - Before Cancer	AC - After Cancer
Type Triple-A+	Type D, on a good day
Worked 10-12 hour days	Work to stay awake 10-12 hours
Living for the dream	Living the dream
Worked for things I could see	Staying alive by the unseen
More money is what I need	Money can't buy life or love
I look good today, and feel so alive	Looking sick every day, I'm glad to be alive
My house payment is due, now what?	Thank you, God, for my house
This steak is overcooked	I am so blessed to taste and enjoy food again
I can't go a day without (whatever)	I made it this far with stage 4 cancer
Others don't respect me	Do I deserve respect?
My wife and family bug me at times	Without my wife and family, I'm not here
What do people think of me?	What do God and my family think of me?
I can do it – I don't need anyone's help	I could not have done it without help
I want what you have	I am content with life and family
Some lowlife scratched my truck	Being able to drive again feels good

My hair is getting gray	Thank God I have hair again
My sex life is great	No sex, but our life is great being together
I have a headache	Aches and pain are "new normal" every day
Look at what I've accomplished	I give credit where credit is due

THE TRUE VALUE OF WORK

I've always liked work. I began working at age 8, and I soon found that I enjoyed the challenge to be good at something. And I liked the rewards! My first job was selling fruit and vegetables to neighbors from my red wagon to make money so I could go fishing. Next, I washed an entire fleet of courier cars on the weekends, and with those earnings I purchased a brand-new .177-caliber pellet rifle. *Oh yeah!* During high school I worked at McDonald's and saved my money for a nice car.

By the age of 19, I was married and working in a restaurant. One day an air conditioning and heating service technician was working up on the restaurant roof. When he was done with the job, I asked him a question on his way out:

"How did you learn to do that?" I asked.

"Went to trade school," he answered.

By that fall, I was working the breakfast and lunch shift from 6 a.m. to 2 p.m. and going to school from 3-11 p.m. I did that routine for nine months. I was hired after my first interview and worked in that trade until age 50.

At one point in my career, I was working full time, 40 hours a week in heating and cooling for a school district during the day, and delivering pizzas until midnight to pay for my out-of-state hunting trips. Long days, hard work and great rewards were a "normal" life for me.

When I was diagnosed with cancer, very likely from the asbestos I'd worked around during my entire career, I had to retire against my will. I found that what I missed most about the job was my interactions with customers. I missed having coffee with them at their kitchen table after having successfully repaired their systems. I missed the fresh baked goods, the jokes, and all the other little things that made owning my own business special.

Before cancer I sacrificed easily those things that now, after cancer, break my heart to miss – school plays, ball games, or just wrestling around on the floor. Now my wife and I are teacher helpers in our grandsons' kindergarten classroom twice a month.

Before cancer I took so many things for granted, all the time thinking I was doing the right thing to earn money to support my family and put something away for retirement, too.

That's important, but it's not all-important. Remember the things that really count. Jobs will come and go – don't let that happen with your family. Family is worth more than anything you'll ever gain with money. It's more important than you'll ever realize until you have six months to live.

Work hard, yes, but not for the worthless things a paycheck can buy. Instead, I'm telling you to invest in the only thing that will always pay back more than you put into it – your family. Please don't wait until cancer or something else takes you captive before you accept and treasure these thoughts.

Take my advice – choose the attitude of "After Captivity." Don't let "Before Captivity" happen to you! Make the right choices that will give you the freedom to enjoy your new investment plan.

I AM WHO I AM

Your friend Jim Morrison is as screwed-up and wacko as ever. Really, not much has changed on that front either before or after cancer. That's because God made me who I am – one of a kind. As I like to say, "The world is safe, since there's only one of me!"

I believe cancer was allowed in my life not to change my personality, but to reconstruct my heart and renew my brainwashed mind. We all get so hung up with the garbage our society dishes out. We are led to believe that if your hair does not glisten just so in the sunlight that no one will notice you. The TV commercial says, "When your hair is together, so are you." *I guess after multiple rounds of chemo, that leaves me out.*

If your handbag is from Target instead of Gucci, then you are of no success. If the car you drive wasn't made the same year that you're living in, then it's junk. And God forbid if you are not on Facebook every minute, take 27 of the right health supplements every morning or have a cell phone that's seven seconds slower than another. (Keep in mind, I'm so old school, I can't even spell "Eye-Pod"!) You are of no importance and left to die.

World, I want a refund, this "mask of deception" is not for me.

With or without all this nonsense, I am who I am. For the most part, I've always lived by what my dad used to say: "You can't please all the people all the time." I have also been told, "God does not make junk." Then why do we risk our lives for a plastic surgeon to make us look better? Have we all become so vain that we cannot accept responsibility for what age, hard work and stupid choices do to us? Can't we accept each other for who we are on the inside instead of what we are supposed to be on the outside?

During the last six months of my dad's life, he finally told me something that he'd never said before. He said he'd become too caught up with keeping up with the world, friends and the image of success he wanted so badly.

When he never achieved success according to popular culture, and his "friends" pulled ahead, he convinced himself that he was a total failure. That's when he looked for help. I wish that he had sought that help from my mom, my sister, my wife or me. We loved him no matter how much or how little he made. We begged to have our husband and father in our lives again. But instead, his new best friend's name was "vodka." Once he turned to alcohol, I watched my father go from a $100,000 annual paycheck as a lumber salesman in 1970 to being a ward of the state and living in a halfway house.

Because of his tragic story, I knew better than to "set myself up" (Daniel 5:23) and get trapped in "captivity" by the "image." I knew firsthand how deceiving it could all become.

But even though I was never as obsessed with image and success as my Dad, the enticement of what this world can offer was quite appealing. That appeal caused me to work out of town for years because the money was very, very good, and allowed my family and me to have what we wanted.

Early one Sunday afternoon, while I was packing to go out of town for the job again, my daughter followed me into the bedroom and asked, "Daddy, how much do you charge per hour to repair a heater?"

"What in the world made you ask that question?" I said.

"I just want to know."

"Sixty-five dollars," I told her.

"Okay" she said. "Goodbye."

It was very late that Friday night by the time I was driving back home. I was in deep thought about my relationship with my children. It bugged the hell out of me that I was not sure how old my daughter was or what grade she was in.

The next morning the kids were excited to see me home for a very short time. My daughter, looking for some daddy time, joined my wife and me at the kitchen table.

She was fumbling with a wad of cash in her hand.

"Honey," I asked, "what's that money for?"

"Daddy, I've been saving my money for a long time, and now I have enough to buy an hour of your time."

Talk about a wakeup call. The next day I drove out of town for my last job there. I'd told my boss I didn't want to work out of town anymore. On my way home the song *"Cat's in the Cradle"* came on the service van's radio.

As Harry Chapin sang that song, every word felt like a blow to my heart.

My child arrived just the other day
He came to the world in the usual way
But there were planes to catch and bills to pay
He learned to walk while I was away
And he was talking 'fore I knew it, and as he grew, he'd say
"I'm gonna be like you, dad. You know I'm gonna be like you"

And the cat's in the cradle and the silver spoon
Little boy blue and the man in the moon
"When you coming home, dad?"
"I don't know when, but we'll get together then, son
You know we'll have a good time then"

My son turned ten just the other day
He said, "Thanks for the ball, dad, come on let's play"
Can you teach me to throw?" I said, "Not today, I got a lot to do"
He said, "That's ok." And he walked away
But his smile never dimmed, and said
"I'm gonna be like him, yeah. You know I'm gonna be like him"

Well, he came home from college just the other day
So much like a man I just had to say
"Son, I'm proud of you. Can you sit for a while?"
He shook his head, and said with a smile
"What I'd really like, dad, is to borrow the car keys
See you later. Can I have them please?"

And the cat's in the cradle and the silver spoon
Little boy blue and the man in the moon
"When you coming home, son?"
"I don't know when, but we'll get together then, dad
You know we'll have a good time then"

I've long since retired, my son's moved away
I called him up just the other day
I said, "I'd like to see you if you don't mind"
He said, "I'd love to, dad, if I can find the time
You see, my new job's a hassle, and the kids have the flu
But it's sure nice talking to you, dad. It's been nice taking to you"

And as I hung up the phone, it occurred to me
He'd grown up just like me
My boy was just like me

And the cat's in the cradle and the silver spoon
Little boy blue and the man in the moon
"When you coming home, son?"
"I don't know when, but we'll get together then, dad
You know we'll have a good time then"

As the song ended, this big tough heating and cooling guy pulled to the side of Highway 5 and I wept uncontrollably. I knew I'd become what I feared most. I had chased the money rabbit down that dark hole of captivity. I needed to climb out, fast.

WHAT'S OUT IS NOT IN

A chemotherapy patient wears many hats, quite literally. When I lost my hair for the first of three times, the cancer center offered me a hat. Without it, the sun felt great in the summer, but come winter, with no hair on your head, it's cold. It was wonderful to find out that volunteers would knit hats and socks for us cancer warriors to wear, and non-profit organizations, along with cancer survivors, would donate wigs and scarves for the women.

God bless you all for helping us cope with the disease. It just feels so good to know others care. Thank you!

I never worried about the loss of all my hair, but most of the women and a few of the men I've met with say it's one of their hardest struggles. They feel exposed and unnatural, but they've learned to cope by realizing it's only temporary. And men and women both have said, "We have bigger fish to fry than worrying about hair." *Amen!*

I remember trying to figure out which new cancer-related problem was more embarrassing: No hair, my flushed red face with huge whitehead pimples, the constant itching everywhere, or having to make bathroom runs, NOW!

Before cancer it was a different story, but now, I don't care what others think. I enjoy each day of life. The change in my appearance on the outside hasn't kept me from fully engaging my life with anyone willing to spend time with me. I am at peace with myself, knowing who I am and what I have accomplished with great help. After cancer,

I am able to focus on inner strength and beauty instead of being freaked out by how others see me.

As a young man, I was always hesitant to try something because I was afraid I would fail and then be belittled, because "a real man could do it." I was constantly told I would never "amount to much." Well, if smoking, drinking, cheating people for ill-gotten gain and looking good but being unfaithful is "amounting to much," then no thanks!

Over the past eight years I have seen many "real men" buried. Cancer eats "real success" for lunch: Money, job titles, power, fame, arrogance, looks and style are no match for this disease.

REAL OR REALITY?

As you know by now, I strongly believe that one of your best weapons against cancer is your attitude.

That includes your attitude toward other cancer warriors. Join the fight together! It takes the right attitude to look past your pain to see the pain of someone else. And you'll need their comfort and advice if you're going to be healed.

This is where your inner reality counts. All the money you have means nothing to a cancer patient on "one of those chemo days." Do you think they care if you're wearing the latest fashions? Does it give them strength to sit up in bed if you're a CEO? The best wealth in a hospital room is an attitude of love and a humbled heart of compassion for a fellow warrior who needs you. Your hand reaching out to help, not to take, will capture their attention and pay dividends for you both. *Trust me! I've been on both sides of this exchange.*

After cancer, I'm aware that I have become much because I have been given much – not from external wealth or beauty, but from an internal attitude of humility. Now I plan to live out my newly extended life with the reality of that dream. I will make time for others with cancer or any captivity. I will radiate genuine success, faith and hope. I will be a witness to my family and to others by being truly happy on the inside and blessed on the outside.

The real rewards in life are the ones nobody sees. The encouragement you offer a dying person will not be broadcast on "Entertainment Tonight." But when you uplift that other person and yourself, you will have an immense flood of joy and satisfaction. Better yet, nobody will know.

The more "real reality" achievements you have, the bigger are the rewards – so much bigger than a new car or a ring. When I drive home after encouraging a fellow cancer warrior, I am on top of the world. I feel like I just won the Super Bowl.

MY SISTER'S DILEMMA

Many years ago, my sister called me to ask for help. She was divorced and was living in a motel room with three kids, no job and no money. Unfortunately, I was still the selfish, hardheaded Jim Morrison of "Before Cancer."

"Sis, you need to make it on your own," I told her. "Every time you're in a jam I don't want you to think you should call your big brother for a handout. I've worked my tail off for everything I have, and it's hard to part with, but I'll help. I'm sending you two hundred bucks. Good luck and call me next week."

Broke and alone, with three young people depending on her for their very existence, she was in the toughest spot of her life. She didn't have a lot of choices left. The one thing she could choose? Her attitude. Her old-fashioned, "common sense" determination helped her climb out of that pit of despair and succeed to this day in the things of life that really count for something.

Even then, some weeks she felt like she would never recover. She was so overwhelmed by the pain and sorrow of her broken family that it seemed easier to die. I felt like that many times with cancer and so will you… *but don't stay there!* Think about the things that matter most. For me, it was thinking about the joy of walking my daughter down the aisle to get married, seeing my son graduate from college, or taking my grandson to his first day of kindergarten.

Day by day, my sister became more confident in herself and her abilities. She broke free from her captivity with a positive attitude that real success is achieved with faith, hope and love.

148

Today my sister is doing well, and so are her kids and their children. It makes me proud to call her Grandma, and for me to be called Uncle Jim. She is rich with what really matters, and you'd never know it. I loved my sis before and after her divorce, but now she's a strong woman who knows her worth and purpose. All the riches this world thinks it offers would never be able to buy what she has on the inside now.

Maybe it's when you have nothing that you gain everything.

MY GREATEST SUCCESS

By now you know that "Before Cancer" I was a Type Triple-A workaholic with an addictive personality. *Go big or go home. I'm in it to win it.* I took this attitude into my battle with cancer – and I think it helped me survive. Over time, cancer and life itself has lessened this intense focus somewhat, yet it still drives my loved ones crazy.

"Jim," my wife tells me, "You're all or nothing."

More than once my kids have said, "Settle down and chill out, Dad, or we're going to call your doctor and have him give you a little dose of chemo to cool your jets."

Even writing this book became an addiction. It took a lot of time away from my family, and after a while, it was all I thought about day and night. I was held "captive" – even by a good thing.

"Before Cancer," my life was all about success. It was all about me. "After Cancer," I still work hard. I do more in a day than some of the healthy people I know, but my entire approach has shifted. That old attitude, thank God, is gone.

"Before Cancer," I believed that I deserved "the good life" since I worked so hard and made it happen. Every thought and moment spent working was fueled by selfish ambition. Work and "success" brought me a real high, but it also held me in captivity. There are many very successful people with my old attitude, but what they often get in return is a sad string of difficulties with marriage, family, unpaid taxes, bankruptcies, broken homes, confused children, fallen church attendance and an unhealthy addiction to something.

With my "old-school" approach (or as my college-educated son puts it, "narrow-minded") and my new "After Cancer" vision, I do not agree any longer with the world's traditional definition of success. I thank cancer for clearing my vision to see what success really means.

A CHANCE TO TELL MY STORY

In 2009, the Kootenai Cancer Center where I received my treatments asked if I would be their spokesman for a new cancer facility. This was my first time to share my story on the "big stage." They put my picture up on billboards along the freeway, in the local newspaper, on TV and on the walls of the hospital. The editor of *CdA Magazine* wrote a feature-length story about me. Wherever I went, people recognized me and knew my story. I was beginning to feel like something special.

As if that wasn't enough, I was asked to speak at the medical center's annual fundraiser. I struggled with how to share something meaningful. I felt the pressure of this very significant occasion, and I just couldn't come up with the right words.

The day of the big speech dawned, and I still had nothing. It was late November, and with archery deer season still open, I headed for the quiet spaces of the forest near my home, my hunting bow in one hand and my pen and writing pad in the other. That night, I would give a speech that right now was just a blank sheet of paper.

I hunkered down in my hunting blind and began to contemplate what I should say. My adventure through cancer land had been overwhelmed with highs and lows. My first impulse was that I should get some real credit for doing all the work and surviving this war. *After all, look at all the recognition and attention I was getting. I must really be something special.*

An hour passed there in the forest, and my pen was still in my pocket. Contemplation had clarified my thoughts. I knew in my heart what I needed to do. I'd discovered this truth long before I had cancer: that success, when combined with pride, is as deadly as can be. I had watched it destroy my father.

I realized that this speech was not about me and about my accomplishments. Instead, it was a God-given moment to share the real things in life with 400 strangers, and to thank those who really deserved the credit for me being here today. With my selfish mind stilled, and my heart ready to share, I pulled out my pen and began to write that evening's speech.

Two hours later, I hadn't seen a deer, but I'd had a very successful hunt in another way: I had my thoughts in order. Later that evening, with speech in hand and a humble attitude in my heart, I stood before a crowd of Coeur d'Alene's elite citizens, nervous but determined to give the performance of my life. This is what I said:

MY SPEECH AT THE FUNDRAISER

"Good evening and welcome to the 21st annual Festival of Trees gala. I want to thank everyone involved in setting me up for this event. This great experience has caused me to do things for women I would never do for my wife… *Wearing a tux in a fashion show? Come on!* I am honored to be able to speak and help the cancer center I love so much.

"Okay, how many of you know a word that starts with F? Raise your hand. Cancer taught me three new 'F' words. Ready?

"First, Faith – being sure of what we hope for and certain of what we do not see. There are many faiths, religions and churches. You have a choice. My name is Jim Morrison and this is my faith: My God holds my life's breath in his hand and He alone controls my destiny. By faith in the name of Jesus this man whom you know and see was made strong.

"Second, Family. You can tell how much courage a family has by how much it takes to discourage them. I want to thank my family for their courage and love, without which I could not have made it this far. Never forget the benefits of family.

"Third, Facilities. I want to personally thank everyone who works with cancer patients at our three great centers. As a cancer patient, it makes a big difference to have confidence in your doctor and cancer center. Over the last five years the wonderful professionals at my cancer center made my family and me very comfortable. That's hard to do when someone you love could die.

"With your help tonight we will fund our brand-new facility with state-of-the-art equipment so cancer patients will become well. The cancer wellness program will be a tremendous boost in spirit for families with cancer of any kind.

"I want you to hear this – cancer is very depressing for the patient and their family. My wife and I had what we called "crybaby days," with both of us overwhelmed by what we were dealing with. With cancer you need people around you that know what to tell you, a mentor if you will.

"I had a mentor, my good friend and hunting partner. He had a year of cancer before I was diagnosed. He had answers to my questions, my fears and depression. I was lucky to have a mentor in the early days of my cancer treatment.

"Some may never have a mentor. That's why we need the cancer wellness program, where every need of the cancer patient and their families will be met. It will change and save lives for your family and others. I want you to know that my sister-in-law is a breast cancer survivor because of our cancer facility. We shared the same doctor and great staff. One family member with cancer is plenty. Two is over the top. We would not be here tonight without the three 'F' words.

"Please support this cause. Please give generously to the cancer wellness program. Let's 'Fund the Need' – I know my family did.

"I'm Jim Morrison and this is my cancer center! Merry Christmas and good night."

MY NIGHT AS A FASHION MODEL

Some would mark the success of that evening by the $90,000 in generous contributions given within ten minutes. But the real measure was the emotional outpouring among us all. Some people cried on my shoulder, hugging and thanking me for the encouragement and unselfish support. I literally ran, yes, a stage 4 lung cancer survivor running table-to-table, thanking the donors from the bottom of my heart. Donor after donor, I felt they were encouraging me even more than I was encouraging them.

That special evening was overwhelming. Those generous donations came in the form of dollars, but none who were in attendance will take one cent with them when they die, including me. But what we will die with is how we felt that night. We all gave up self for the greater good. We all did our part to close the curtain on this killer with no encore. *Amen!*

What could top that experience?

It happened two nights later, when my four-year-old grandson, "Mr. B", and I walked together in the evening fashion show featuring cancer survivors. We were fully decked out in Christmas-themed tuxedos – looking good and feeling good! Through the curtain and down the walkway we went, to a standing ovation that still brings tears to my eyes to remember it. There were no words to describe this very precious moment in time with my grandson, who by all odds I was never supposed to meet.

My grandson captivated that crowd. As he trotted down the runway, he invented his now-famous "double-handed wave," which drew a joyful roar from the audience. He was having the time of his young life.

For my part, I was crying so hard I could hardly see the runway through my tears. As I looked down to the table with my wonderful family and friends, and saw the happiness of my grandson, even more tears came flowing. I was struck by the absolute miracle of the moment.

To be alive and to walk the runway that night was a testimony to the power of faith, family and all the great professionals who treated me in our outstanding facilities. It was a living, breathing example of what these things can achieve when they work together for good.

Today, if you gave me a choice of "Before Cancer" or "After Cancer;" believe it or not, I would choose the life I've learned after cancer. I'm now truly successful with things that have real meaning. All my life I'd searched for success, and at the very end of me, success was there.

I have the love and respect of my children and grandchildren. I am still married to the only women I would ever want to spend my life with. For more than forty years she's been there for me. She's been my anchor so I would not drift too far. She was loyal to me throughout my addiction and recovery, and my very faithful helper during my war with cancer.

Faith, family, hope, love and compassion, that's what makes us a success together. The true happiness we have today is something I wish for you, my friend.

Sometimes, you can only find it after the captivity of something like cancer leads you to the end of yourself.

Warrior Words

I remember it all beginning with Dad going to the ER after a hunting trip with Jeff and just not feeling well. I remember being at work and talking to him about how he was feeling and laughing to myself that he sounded like one of my congestive heart failure patients. About a week later it was not so funny anymore, since he was a congestive heart failure patient; not because of a bad heart, but due to a liter of bloody fluid on his heart.

As a nurse and a daughter I find it hard to wear only one of those hats. At times through all of this I wished I were only a daughter and not the nurse who knew what the doctors were not saying. I felt the most pressure from Mom who would look at me when we were talking to the doctors to see my reaction. It was these times I really wanted to take off my nurse hat and just be a daughter. Then on the other hand I was so very thankful to be a nurse to know what the doctors were not saying and to know what was serious and just part of it.

Looking back now that pressure I was under as a nurse/daughter has made me the nurse I am today to be able to work in the Cardiac Intensive Care Unit and know the other side of my job. When I was working out at Curves when Mom came and got me back to the hospital for Dad's gallbladder surgery. I do not remember much of the waiting, since at this time we knew nothing more than a poor HIDA scan result.

The next day, it all began. Why could Dad not be weaned off the oxygen? Why the pain in his calf when we got him up to the bathroom after a gallbladder surgery? What was going on? The general surgeon wanted answers, too. And the chest CT was just what he needed. When the pace of the nurses and doctors pick up, whether you're medical trained or not, you know something is not right. Off to ICU, and for no reason except God wanted me there, I was in the ICU as they were hooking Dad up to the monitors. I remember our family doctor being at the desk looking over the CT when the blood pressure cuff went off and Dad's blood pressure was not right. I asked Dad how he was feeling and when the answer was "a lot of pressure" on his chest, I knew it was not good.

I went to the nurse station, saw the fear in our primary doctor's eyes, and left the ICU holding my breath, waiting to hear a code blue called to Dad's room. I remember feeling numb to the situation and telling Mom "he will be fine." I have no idea how much time passed before the doctors came into that room to tell us that they had just pulled a total of three liters of fluid out of his chest. Oh, and by the way, it was all bloody. Oh boy, I thought. Then of course it was Friday night, and pathology would not be done until Monday. I think that was the longest weekend on record. I traded shifts with him in his ICU room, or in the waiting room with a LOT of friends and family. Who knew Dad was so popular? Then came Monday morning, and we heard the news from the oncologist.

A lot of things went though my mind while Dad was in the hospital for the first two weeks. Would I erase or keep his cell phone number in my phone just to call sometimes to hear his message? Who would walk me down the aisle for my wedding that summer? Would my kids ever know him? How would we take care of Mom?

One day when I could not take the sights and sounds of the ICU anymore, I walked the halls of the hospital and came upon the chapel. I went in and found myself the only one there. So to my knees I fell and knew in my heart I was not going to get through this without help. As I prayed I felt less anxious and a little more able to focus.

That night I had some friends over. I was crying about it when one of my friends looked at me and said "Why are you burying him before he is dead?" From then on, I knew it was okay, even though we still had a long road to go. I could be a nurse and a daughter and be able to withstand the pressure of both.

I got married, have two boys that adore their "Papa," and still have my Dad around who I can be a nurse and daughter to. We had a couple surgeries, a lot of chemotherapy, a lot of PET scans, doctor visits, some pretty bad times with the chemotherapy, but here we are today to tell them. I have never once asked God why. I do not think at the time I knew the answer, but looking back now, this has been such a blessing. It brought me back to my Christian walk, and gave me life lessons that cannot be taught in a classroom on how to be both a nurse AND a daughter.

–Kym Hamby, R.N.
Jim's daughter

After my father's chemotherapy, when they got the cancer under control, we got the opportunity to go hunting 3-4 days a week. We were only able to do this by the power of God. We had the best duck and goose hunting season that anyone could ever have. Yeah, we filled our limit almost every day, but that wasn't the best part. The best part was that I got to see another one of God's sunrises with my father every morning that we shared in the hunting blind. We can thank the Lord for my father's recovery from cancer. I guess God wasn't done with him just yet. He has many more missions to carry out as a HOLY SOLDIER. From the day he was able to get up and spread the word of the Lord, that is just what he did. I don't see that coming to an end anytime soon. Praise God for that. There are many more seasons to come, thanks to the healing hands of the Lord.

God Bless,

–Jeff Morrison
Jim's son

CHAPTER 9
Through Thick and Thin

At the very beginning of my cancer, lying there scared, angry and depressed in my hospital bed, I set a simple goal for myself – to live for one more hour.

When I saw that I had stayed alive that hour, I would set a higher mark of staying alive for two whole hours.

At first I was afraid to fall asleep, not knowing what the cancer could do to me during the night. All my life, I'd never given a thought to whether I'd wake up the next morning or not. As hours became weeks, I grew less afraid of the act of going to sleep, since by then I had witnessed many new sunrises through my hospital window.

It's amazing what hope a sunrise can bring.

I am happy to tell you that I have seen many more sunrises since that dark January day I was diagnosed.

I have watched the sun come up on the day of my sweet daughter's wedding and the birth of my grandsons. I have felt the sun shine on my son's fine graduation. With my high school sweetheart, I've witnessed the sunrise from the beach in Tahiti, our tropical dream for 40 years of marriage finally come true. And I have seen the sun light up the wilderness sky on those beloved hunting trips I feared would never, ever come again. Most recently, I have lived to stand up and speak at my boy's wedding ceremony. And what an incredible feeling that was.

The day before the wedding, excitement ran high. The outdoor setting was beautifully decorated, and my boy, Jeff, and his bride-to-be, Stephanie James, were eager for the ceremony. I left the hubbub behind and walked to my favorite quiet place in the woods. I paused to reflect.

It all came flooding back. How much terror had filled my first night in the ICU with just six months to live. How helpless, scared and utterly overwhelmed I felt. How I knew I would not be around much longer for my family. The fact that at 50, I felt very much cheated by my cancer. How angry I was to have my life cut short. How much I would miss. How my future was gone.

As you've read in this book, I changed my attitude. I began seeing each act of survival as a new goal. My future was each milestone in the lives of those I loved.

Along the way, cancer gave me a true appreciation for life. Now I cherish every breath, every hug from my grandsons and every goodnight kiss from my wife. Cancer gave me back life's true meaning, and for that I will always be grateful.

Tomorrow is a powerful word. There were many days I'd questioned whether I'd live until tomorrow, and now tomorrow held the promise of my boy's wedding. Waking up tomorrow means you've beaten your captivity one more day.

Tomorrow, I was ready to stand up at that wedding and say a word – okay, you know me better than that – maybe quite a few words. And here are exactly those words I spoke that day, at a wedding I shouldn't have lived long enough to attend:

MY SPEECH AT MY SON'S WEDDING

"Good evening everyone, and thank you for being here to celebrate this most sacred time for two very special people. When your children get married it is always a special, joyous and sometimes tearful occasion, with family and friends gathered to celebrate one of God's true blessings – marriage. This union also brings together families and starts new relationships. I must say that Stephanie's "James gang" is wonderful. At this point, though, I'm still not sure who are the in-laws or the outlaws!

"Today is more than a special day for me – today is a miracle. This evening is allowed by God's unmerited grace for me to share with my family and friends. On January 13, 2004, I was given six months to live due to work-related stage 4 lung cancer. My first goal was to be at my daughter's wedding, and Kym and Jimmy were married in July of 2004. By undeserved favor I was there. My next goal was to witness the births of my grandsons, Byron and Carter, a blessing I will always cherish and be grateful for.

"For me to attend Jeff's graduation in May of 2007 from the University of Idaho made me so proud of my son. He made me feel special by saying: 'Jimbo, through all the college and cancer, we are sharing this special day together. We have accomplished our goals against all odds.'

"And here today, July 23, 2011, six and half years later, another impossible goal has been reached. I am here to witness my son be married to my wonderful daughter-in-law, Stephanie. Undeserved grace is the power in which this sinner stands before you all today.

"That same God tells us in Proverbs 18, verse 22, "He who finds a wife finds what is good and receives favor from the Lord." This verse states that it is good to be married. Today's emphasis on individual freedom is misguided. God created marriage for our enjoyment and He pronounced it good.

"Today, my son, you take on the responsibility of being the spiritual leader in your home. I am so blessed to be here and witness my Jeff take on his new mission. With a loving wife on one side and God's favor on the other, all things are possible. I know!

"Jeff and Stephanie, I'd like to share this wisdom, from 39 years of marriage and the Bible:

Marriage is God's idea.

Commitment is essential to a successful marriage.

Marriage holds times of great joy and sadness.

Unfaithfulness breaks the bond of trust.

Marriage is permanent. Ideally only death should dissolve marriage.

Jeff, I have warned Stephanie; he's yours now, no refund, no return,

and no exchange.
And finally the good stuff – romance is important!
Marriage creates the best environment for raising children.

"Get the hint? My newest goal is to meet my new granddaughter someday. And maybe some more grandsons to carry on the Morrison name! Either way, I am so proud of Jeff and the honor he has brought to our name. I am so proud to have my Stephanie share our name. Today my son, you take on a wife and that is good. Stephanie, today you take on a husband and that is good. Jeff and Stephanie, today you become as one and that is good.

"Today, I thank God again for extending my life to accomplish this most impossible, important goal. And for allowing me this day against all odds, I love you both, thank you."

As I looked out at those wonderful faces, not an eye was dry. Everyone knew they had just seen something that should never have been. Once again, I had learned that the most wonderful things in life are the things you earn by defying the odds, and by sharing those precious moments with others.

And now, I take the center floor with my son's wife. Wow. The music hasn't started and yet I'm crying anyway. I'm hugging her tight, overwhelmed by what this means. How grateful I am to still be alive for this dance.

You can beat the odds. You can keep hope before you. You can believe in things yet unseen. You can live to dance that most important dance.

My dear friend, I want you to find the faith, family and facilities you need to live.

And then, I want you to do the hardest, most important part:

I want you to survive just one more hour.

I need you to survive that one more hour so that someday soon, you will live to see the things that you could only dream.

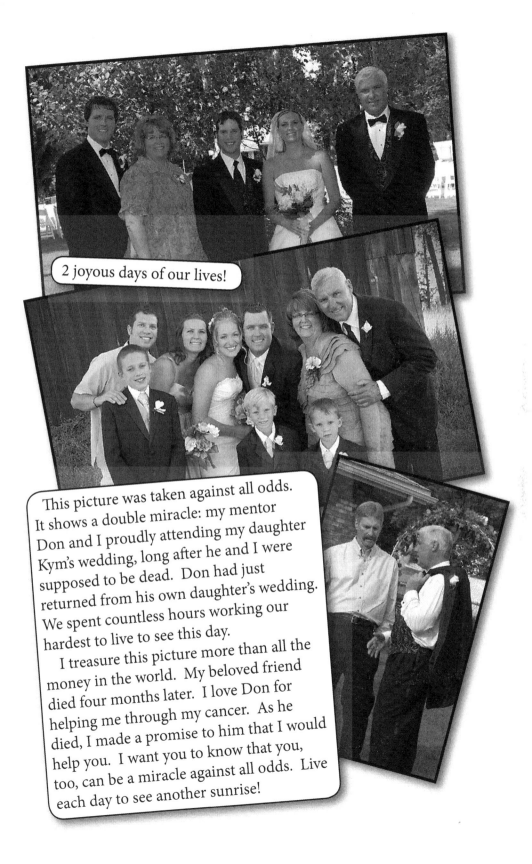

2 joyous days of our lives!

This picture was taken against all odds. It shows a double miracle: my mentor Don and I proudly attending my daughter Kym's wedding, long after he and I were supposed to be dead. Don had just returned from his own daughter's wedding. We spent countless hours working our hardest to live to see this day.

I treasure this picture more than all the money in the world. My beloved friend died four months later. I love Don for helping me through my cancer. As he died, I made a promise to him that I would help you. I want you to know that you, too, can be a miracle against all odds. Live each day to see another sunrise!

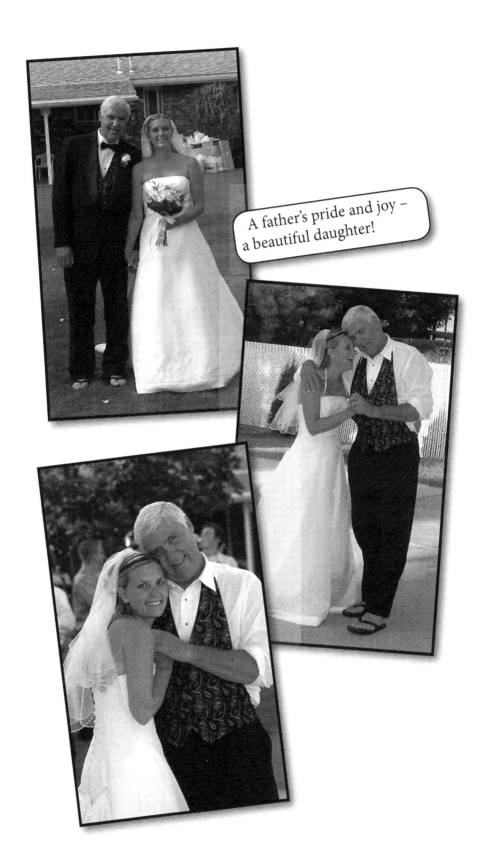

A father's pride and joy – a beautiful daughter!

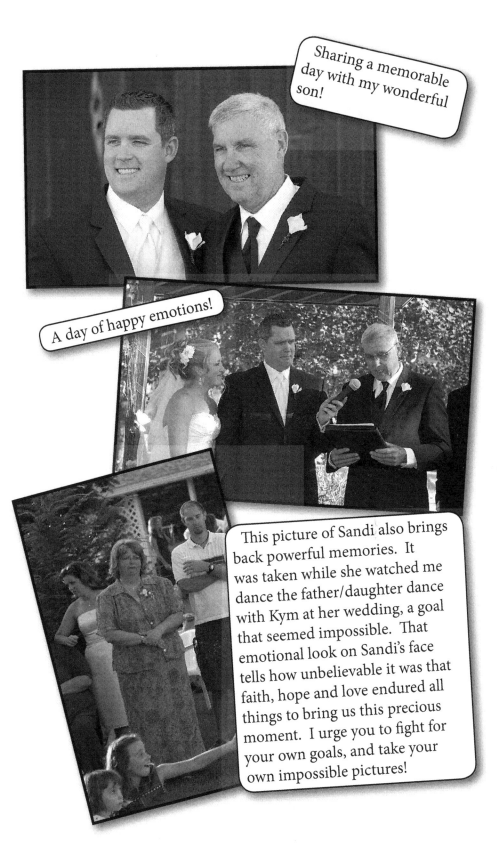

Sharing a memorable day with my wonderful son!

A day of happy emotions!

This picture of Sandi also brings back powerful memories. It was taken while she watched me dance the father/daughter dance with Kym at her wedding, a goal that seemed impossible. That emotional look on Sandi's face tells how unbelievable it was that faith, hope and love endured all things to bring us this precious moment. I urge you to fight for your own goals, and take your own impossible pictures!

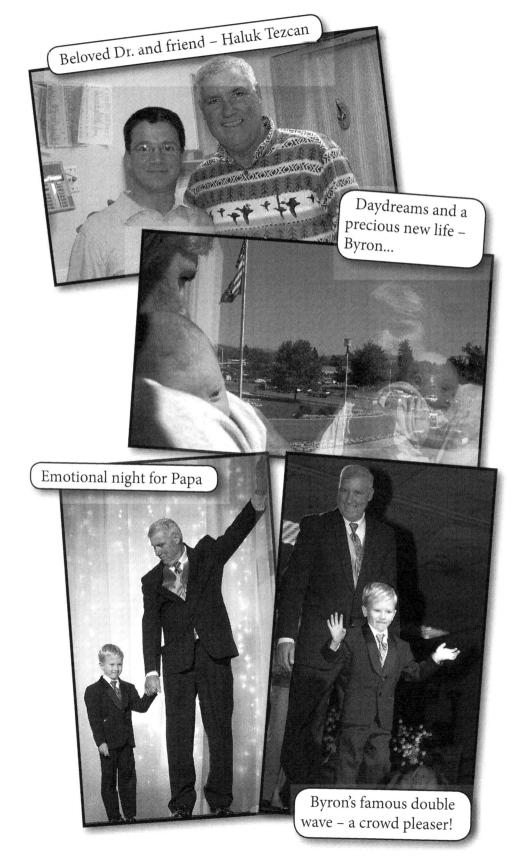

Beloved Dr. and friend – Haluk Tezcan

Daydreams and a precious new life – Byron...

Emotional night for Papa

Byron's famous double wave – a crowd pleaser!

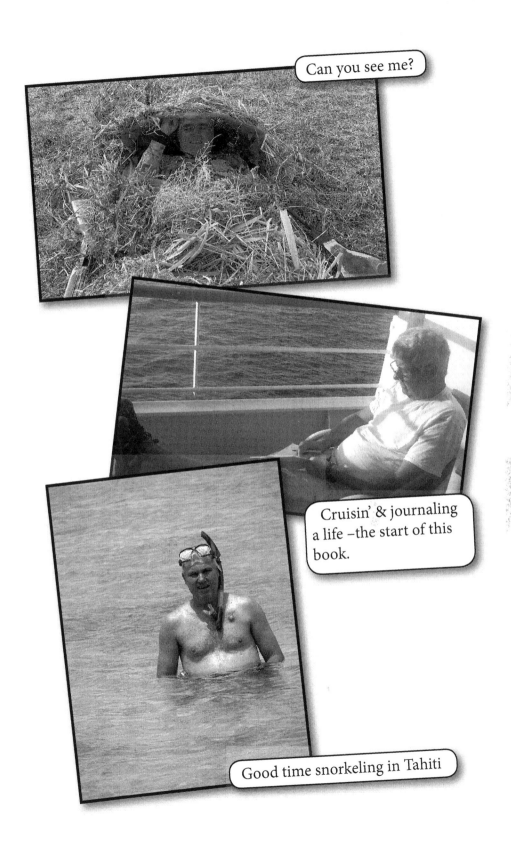

Can you see me?

Cruisin' & journaling a life –the start of this book.

Good time snorkeling in Tahiti

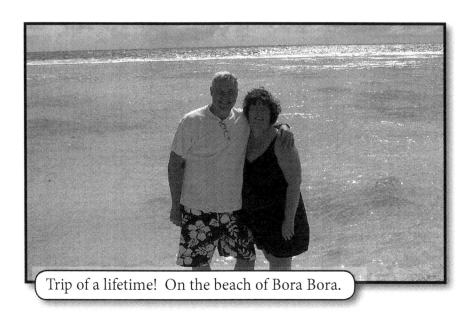

Trip of a lifetime! On the beach of Bora Bora.

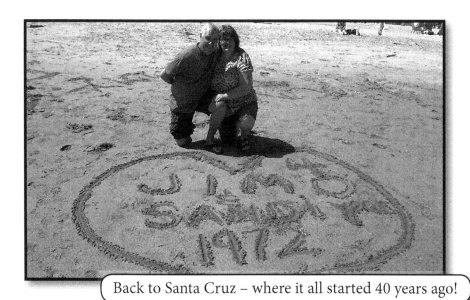

Back to Santa Cruz – where it all started 40 years ago!

In The End It All Begins

Well there it is…my true-life story.

Did this book encourage you? Then please encourage someone else. Share your story and your time with them. Give them a copy of this book.

I would like to hear your story, too. Please e-mail me, and I will do my best to answer.

If I don't answer right away, it might be because I'm at another grandkid's birth, in the hospital room with someone who needs me, taking time to spend with my wife and family, or out hunting in the wild places I love best.

I would love to hear about your goals – and tell you about my latest ones, too.

I love you fellow cancer warrior,

Jim Morrison
toseeanothersunrise@gmail.com

A percentage of the proceeds from the sale of this book go directly to Cancer Center – Kootenai Health Foundation.

40609019R00103

Made in the USA
Middletown, DE
17 February 2017